This book is dedicated to my wonderful wife, Bev, who wholeheartedly supported me through this whole journey. And to my beautiful daughters, Laura, Sarah, Michelle, and Jenny, who, along with their husbands, Marc, Steve, Jesse, and Alvin, have collectively provided me with eleven wonderful grandchildren.

a slimmer You

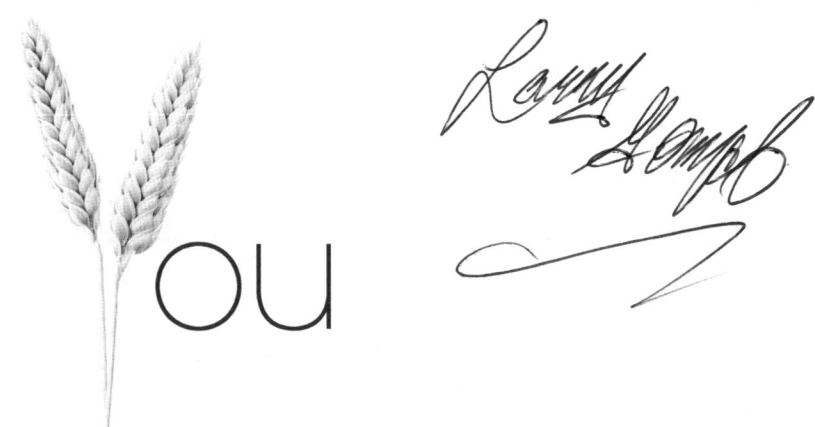

A NATURAL WAY TO LOSE WEIGHT

BY LARRY GOMPF

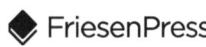 FriesenPress

One Printers Way
Altona, MB R0G 0B0
Canada

www.friesenpress.com

Copyright © 2022 by Larry Gompf
First Edition — 2022

All rights reserved.

No part of this publication may be reproduced in any form, or by any means, electronic or mechanical, including photocopying, recording, or any information browsing, storage, or retrieval system, without permission in writing from FriesenPress.

ISBN
978-1-03-913672-4 (Hardcover)
978-1-03-913671-7 (Paperback)
978-1-03-913673-1 (eBook)

1. HEALTH & FITNESS, WEIGHT LOSS

Distributed to the trade by The Ingram Book Company

TABLE OF CONTENTS

Chapter 1
    Introduction 11

Chapter 2
    What Does a Healthy Person Look Like? 15

Chapter 3
    Motivation and Inspiration 21

Chapter 4
    Eat Less 27

Chapter 5
    The Goal 31

Chapter 6
    Fad Diets Don't Work 37

Chapter 7
    The Scales 43

Chapter 8
    Getting Fit 49

Chapter 9
    Staying Fit 55

Chapter 10
    The Value of Core Strength 63

Chapter 11
    How Bad is Belly Fat? 67

Chapter 12
    We Aren't Created Equal 73

Chapter 13
    The Value of Proper Nutrition 79

Chapter 14
    Three Renegades of Processed Food 85

Chapter 15
    Benefits of a Dog 93

Chapter 16
    How Fit is the Retired Farmer? 99

Chapter 17
    Living For Your Grandkids 105

Chapter 18
    Living to be 110 111

Chapter 19
    See Say Safety 117

Chapter 20
    Listen to the Music 123

Chapter 21
    Mental Fitness 129

Chapter 22
    Compressed Morbidity 137

Chapter 23
    The Other Side of the Coin 143

Chapter 24
    IF 151

Afterword: 159

About the Author 163

This is ultimately a book about weight loss. That's how it started out. But it's more than a book about shedding weight and keeping it off. It really is a combination of doing the right things with your life to ensure a healthy lifestyle. It starts with a determination to lose weight in the most natural way you can imagine. And that intertwines with a positive attitude, eating healthy food combined with a certain level of physical fitness. It's tied to a curious and active mind that might help keep you going far into your senior years. Isn't that what we all want for ourselves? But it's not just about what *we* want, because if you listen to your sons and daughters (those who care most about you), it's what *they* want for you, as well. They want you to be able to play with your grandchildren and lift them up and get down on the floor and connect with them. And, who knows, if you strike the right balance of happy living, maybe you'll be able to play and lift and get down on the floor with your great-grandchildren, as well. That's what creates a spark for your future life. In the end, you'll be able to say it certainly was all worth it. It isn't rocket science, but the best part is that *you* can start today. It's that easy. And I know that if I can do it by following a few rules outlined in this book, then *you* should be able to do so, as well. And you'll be on *your* way to *A Slimmer You*. Good luck with your own journey. My journey started when I saw a profile picture of myself that I didn't like.

—Larry Gompf

"Thanks to Renee Friesen for kindly photographing a number of the pictures in this book."

CHAPTER 1
Introduction

The first thing I want you to know as you read this book is who I am. I was born in the Virden hospital in the southwest part of the province of Manitoba, smack in the centre of Canada. I grew up on a mixed farm that would be considered small by today's standards but was average or bigger back then, being a section in size. I loved the farm and grew up in ordinary circumstances. My family consisted of a sister, Marlene, who is the oldest, and two older brothers, Garnet and Karl. There were four of us in four years, so you know it was busy times around our farm. Unfortunately, Garnet passed away on July 17, 2020, following a struggle with cancer.

I remember the day my dad (George) came home with a new Minneapolis Moline U tractor and I crawled over and under that tractor and, to this day, I can still smell the fresh paint emanating from that tractor. That was in the early 1950s and, later, Dad purchased a Massey Harris 21 A combine. Again, I was very excited to see that combine arrive. I got to drive it on my own when I was twelve. That was so exciting.

My siblings and I attended a one-room local school (Harvey) that was two miles from our yard. We went there by horse and buggy, horse and sleigh, or by riding our bicycles until I was in Grade 6. Then Harvey school closed forever and we went to school in the town of Oak Lake. You might say that I had a very normal rural upbringing. For a few years when I was an early teen, I raised and looked after 100 turkeys, which I sold around the neighbourhood. I did that for a few years until I discovered girls and then my life's ambitions changed. No time for turkeys then.

On the farm, a person is always active, so as a result, I could eat as much food as I wanted to. Food that was always fresh or canned for the winter months. Because my mother (Evelyn) was a great cook, there was never a shortage of homemade bread, cakes, or delicious pies of all kinds. I could snack between meals and there was no problem getting rid of any extra calories I consumed. When I left home, I weighed 125 pounds on a five-foot-ten-inch frame. I simply burned off any extra calories from eating lots of food, which included second helpings and, always, desserts.

Eventually, I went off to the University of Manitoba to get a degree in Agriculture. Upon graduation, I started to work in the agricultural chemical industry. However, in the late 1970's and early 80's I took time out to try my hand at grain farming in the Birtle/Isabella area of Manitoba. I wasn't as successful at the business of farming as my neighbours were but I certainly met some wonderful people from that area of the province.

Back in the ag chem industry, over time I became more sedentary and a lot less active. And my job required me to be on the road a lot. That meant many meals at a variety of restaurants in small towns and in the cities across Manitoba and Saskatchewan and some in Alberta. The food was good and was often accompanied by a beer or two.

So, you can guess what started to happen to me! That's right, I gradually gained weight. It was subtle and you could say that I never even noticed what was happening and I didn't really care. Life went on.

Here, I have to caution you, the reader, that I am not in the medical field, I do not have a background in nutrition, and I am not a personal trainer. I wrote this book as an ordinary person, like you, who gained more weight than what was needed for someone of my age and body stature. Over time, I got rid of those extra pounds through what I call the most natural way to lose weight. I lost weight even though I continued to eat all the foods I've always loved to eat. And that includes desserts, which I still enjoy to this very day. I'm hoping that you enjoy reading about my weight-loss journey, which started twelve years ago, in 2010. It took me three years to reach my final weight-loss goal and I've kept off the unneeded pounds for over nine years. I believe I have a story that is worth sharing with you. And I hope it inspires you to try to shed pounds that you don't need and to do it safely and slowly.

The weight I had gained did not put me into the category of being obese, but I knew I was carrying too much weight although I didn't think too much about it at the time. After all, I was a functioning middle-aged person who believed that the look I had was normal. But you all know what happens when, over time, you eat too many burgers—combined with fries, of course, and sometimes covered in gravy. Or you have the special of the day, which often means meat and mashed potatoes slathered with gravy once again. This is often followed by dessert, which might be a piece of pie or cake accompanied by ice cream. And numerous times there would be a milkshake thrown in for good measure. After regularly bolting down that type of meal, I'd be back in the vehicle and driving to the next location. The calories from those lunches just kept adding up over time. If it was a buffet, then total calories consumed were even higher.

But I wasn't quite as bad as some of the folks I'd see lining up for meals at all-you-can-eat buffets. I observed many who were already overweight and they'd load up their plate as if it were their last meal. And then, because it was a buffet, they'd load it up by at least another half and pitch in for desserts, as well. Then they'd crawl back into their vehicle and head off down the highway. For many, that was their daily routine. My goodness, they consumed a lot of extra calories, which you know were headed straight to their waistlines.

a slimmer you

But I shouldn't have been so smug. When I looked at the picture of me taken by my friend Jim Ellis, in 2009, I thought I looked pregnant. I know that many people are comfortable with that look, but for me, I didn't like what I saw. So right then I decided to try to shed some of the extra weight I was seeing on the scale. I didn't want to join any of the available weight-loss groups and I certainly did not want to go on any crash diets. Nor did I want to consume un-needed supplements or protein shakes that all promised weight loss. I rationalized that the pregnant-looking belly had to be from consuming more food than I needed, which of course meant too many calories. And I realized that it was happening every day. So, I decided to adjust my intake of food. I was determined to try to eat mainly healthy foods, to watch closely any progress I might be making, and to make sure I got some form of exercise. Along the way I made a few other small changes and I became determined to stick to my game plan. And for me, it worked. It was a slow process but I am convinced that if it takes several years to add extra weight to your body then you must lose it slowly. I was never interested in the "lose-weight-quickly" mantra that many diets were claiming. I was determined to follow my plan and see if it would work for me.

When you choose to lose weight slowly it's all about paying attention. It is a slow progression but involves all or most of the little steps I advocate in this book. If you do some of them or manage to follow all of my suggestions, you'll see progress over time with your own program. Again, I want to emphasize that the progress will be slow and it does require some level of will power and resolve in order to get started and to stick with the plan once you begin.

I decided to weigh myself every morning before showering. That's the time of day when you will weigh the least. There is more about this in the chapter on using the scale and you'll find that its regular use enabled me to spot the trends of gaining or losing weight and to adjust accordingly.

During my weight-loss period, I learned to gauge when I was eating too much and when I needed to cut back. That is a major key if you plan to lose weight and get down to a natural weight for your body size. And when it comes to exercising, I realized that I did not need to "go nuts" and work out like crazy to start to lose weight. I'm convinced that is the wrong way for an older person to go about losing weight. However, it may be just right for someone a lot younger. High-level aerobic training may work for a few older folks, but really most of us just want or need a level of exercise that fits our age and lifestyle. We are all still conscious of how we look and we work hard to display an image of ourselves to the outside world. There's nothing wrong with that, but I believe it's also important to think about how we feel on the inside. Many folks suffer from aches and pains every day. And that could be joint pain (knee and hip are very common), arthritic pain, or back pain. Some people have osteoporosis and many suffer from other physical ailments. You know that some of these health problems exist because people continue to carry more weight than they need.

Another method of controlling weight is to pay to have meals delivered to your door. Those types of plans can work for you, as they are all about dealing with portion size. If they only deliver the amount of food you need for losing or maintaining weight, then it will work. But why not do the same thing in your own kitchen? You can control your own portion size and you know how much salt, sugar, or fat is in your meal. And of course, meals delivered to your door will cost more than meals you prepare yourself.

Processed meals that you buy and heat up are huge culprits for gaining weight. They do nothing for a weight-loss program. They often are loaded with too many calories and that will have the opposite effect of what you are seeking.

As you've gathered, I'm a fan of fresh food. Good, wholesome foods for centuries have provided all the nutrients that a person needs. Now we are faced with so many choices. Advertising everywhere tries to convince us that we need to complement our food intake with all different types of supplements. They can be costly and if you are eating properly anyway, then you shouldn't need them.

I've also discovered a side benefit to having reduced my weight. Every once in a while, I would experience acid reflux or GERD, as it is commonly called. The medical term for this unpleasant condition is gastroesophageal reflux disease.

I think many people have experienced GERD and it happens when acid comes back up into your mouth. It tastes awful and sometimes leaves your throat feeling sore after the experience. Well, I'm pleased to report that, since I have gotten rid of those extra pounds, acid reflux happens only once or twice a year instead of semi-frequently, like it used to. I say good riddance. Some folks take a prescription drug to control GERD, but I've found that even though I was headed in that direction, it's something I no longer have to consider. Also, I've noticed that my supply of Tums in the medicine cabinet doesn't disappear as fast as it did at one time.

I decided to adjust my intake of food and I was determined to try to eat mainly healthy foods.

TIPS FROM CHAPTER 1:

1. Eat healthy food.

2. Keep track of your weight.

3. Lose weight slowly—no quick-loss diets.

CHAPTER 2
What Does a Healthy Person Look Like?

Have you ever been in a room where a very confident person walks in and the conversation stops? These people seem to suck the oxygen right out of the room. Attention is diverted to them and they seem to be surrounded by admirers. People want to talk to them and share in what they have to say. This observation does not just refer to celebrities or sports heroes, but to ordinary folks who carry themselves with an air of confidence. They don't have a secret, but they are invariably in good health, fit, and dressed for the occasion. What is it that makes them different from the rest of the crowd? Well, it's not just their appearance. They enter a room with confidence and they portray a person who is in full control of themselves. Of course, we are curious to know what sets these people apart from the rest of us.

When a person looks good, they feel good and they carry themselves with confidence. And that boils down to a look and a feel of a positive attitude. There are many people—friends, neighbours, and even some relatives—who don't necessarily suck the air out of the room but do command attention because of who they are and how they carry themselves. And it almost always starts with a positive attitude. It works for them and these folks always approach each day, and life in general, with an attitude that the cup is half full. There is always something positive about a rainy day that washes out a planned picnic. "The crops can use a good drink," or "The lake was getting low and my floating dock was riding too low in the water."

A healthy person has a strong desire to engage with people. Conversation is easy for them and if you look at them as they talk to others, they are always interested in what others are saying. They don't only want to tell their own story but they are genuinely interested in what the people around them are up to as well. And they stay engaged with the conversation. There will be laughter that punctuates the conversation and there will be plenty of smiles.

There's an old saying that goes like this, "You are the average of the 5 people who you spend the most time with." If you are the average, then there is someone in that group who is the most above average. They may not know that they stand out but you surely do notice. And you do not want to fall below that average. But the one who is at the top of the group is the one you like and want to gravitate towards. Why? Because they boost you up and help you to be a more confident and cheery self. You naturally want to be in their camp. If they help to make you a better person, then people will want to be around you and benefit from the positive attitude that you have to offer.

When you look around, it is easy to see who you would like to associate with. Isn't it better to be with folks who portray the confidence of a person with a healthy outlook about life than someone who is a negative-nelly? You don't want to be around someone who sees the glass as half-empty. They drag you down and, the next thing you know, you might start agreeing with their point of view. It's best to avoid these folks and surround yourself with people who have a happier outlook on life.

When I decided to lose weight, I wanted to look slimmer than I was when I looked at that picture Jim took, in which I looked pregnant. Imagine! I couldn't help but think to myself: *What man is happy knowing he looks pregnant?* Or: *What am I doing carrying extra fat that I don't need?* So, I started my journey to lose weight and, as I mentioned before, I didn't want to lose the extra fat too quickly. I also didn't want to give up eating the wholesome, healthy food that I had always eaten. Including desserts. By reducing my daily intake of food, I was able to lose five pounds over a period of time. Back then, I had no set goals of where I wanted to be. I just wanted to lose weight. And it worked. *But, if I can lose five pounds I don't need, then why not keep doing what I was doing?* So, I kept my regimen going and, over time, maybe two years or so, I shed fifteen pounds. By this time, I was feeling fairly smug. I had shed all this weight I didn't need to be carrying and I'd done it without running marathons every day, being a gym rat, or going on a strict diet. I did it in a way that I thought was natural for me (eating everything I've ever eaten) and losing weight slowly. That was my aim. No supplements, protein shakes, or pills designed to clean the toxins out of my system or otherwise cleanse my guts. I was proud and happy with myself until I checked what a man my age and height should weigh. The chart I was able to find on the internet told me I still needed to lose another eleven pounds. What?

I questioned myself. *How can I make this happen?* The easy part was to decide to continue doing what I had been doing. The most difficult part of the equation was to shed those last eleven pounds. But I kept my regimen going, and after three years from when I'd started, I got down to what I consider a natural or ideal weight for me. It meant a new wardrobe for me—but that was the pleasant part of dropping the weight. The real bonus was to feel better about myself. I had more energy and I knew my heart wasn't pumping so hard, circulating blood to areas of my body that were no longer there. And all of a sudden, I realized that I was able to accomplish more than when I was carrying extra weight. Also, like a miracle, some of the things that I was already doing just seemed to be easier. And I felt really good about these accomplishments.

Also, I looked good to my four daughters, Laura, Sarah, Michelle, and Jenny, who are all pleased with the progress I've made. They want me to be around for a long time yet. They want me to enjoy the grandchildren they've brought into the world and to continue to mentor and teach them. And I want to be around for them. The future looks brighter for me because I decided to make a few small adjustments to my lifestyle.

I have a friend who keeps doing new things. He is one of the people I know who has a very positive outlook on life. He listens to what I have to say when he converses with me and he always has a smile and a kind word. He is a successful businessman who must have a great rapport with his employees because he has grown his business over the years and has managed to surround himself with good staff. And, to me, he appears to be very fit. He looks as if he hasn't gained any extra weight over the years.

What's his secret? I know that he has just been himself over these many years. A very positive person. He has managed to stay young in manner and appearance (with the odd grey hair) and portrays a demeanour of always being curious about what is going on around him. That attitude enables him to look ahead and not look back. He has viewed setbacks in his life and business as opportunities to be a better businessman and a better person.

So, you would think that a successful businessman would sit on his laurels and accept the rest of his life in relaxation. Nope! That's not his style. He continuously looks for more opportunities and doesn't shrink from trying something that *could* be successful. That's just who he is. He's definitely someone to look up to and admire. Is he wearing out? I don't think so. He has a wonderful way of balancing workplace demands with other worldly and personal demands of his life. And if you were to ask him, I know he would say that he wouldn't have it any other way. He's happy in his own skin and would take on a new project in a heartbeat if he assessed it and thought it would make sense to tackle and add to his business portfolio.

Overall, what is his secret? It appears to be to stay fit, to stay engaged, to stay curious, to keep smiling, to enjoy every day with a positive attitude, and to take on more responsibilities, if they make sense. If those are his secrets to success, then he makes it look easy. Too bad everyone wasn't so blessed!

But you, too, can reach that stage if you start to make a few small changes in your life. And the first change might be to adopt a positive attitude. Try seeing the cup as half full more often. You'll find that it's easier than you thought and you'll be happier with yourself in the end.

Along with a new attitude, you'll want to look better as well. And this new beginning starts with a desire to shed some unneeded pounds. To me, losing weight slowly was very important. It took a life-time to put on that extra weight, so you have to be patient as you take your time to lose it. It isn't easy but I am living proof that it can work. Twelve years ago, I decided I wanted to shed extra pounds, and it took me three years to do it and for over nine years I've kept it off. And to me, that is the secret. Not really the secret, I want to profess. Perhaps instead, it should be called the "not-so-secret" guide to success. Why? Because all the ways that helped *me* lose weight are there in front of you. When you decide it is time to get started, you'll find that this method might work for you, too.

And that means no fad diets, no extra supplements, no protein shakes, and, least of all, no desire to lose weight *quickly*. Those methods create a yoyo effect on your body whereby you lose weight fast, look good for a while, and then gain the weight back again. And the cycle starts over again. I don't believe these methods are healthy for anyone's well-being. It drives me crazy to see magazines at food store checkouts declaring in bold titles that you can lose twenty-four pounds in a week if you just follow this newly discovered Soup Diet or whatever the diet of the day is. Every week or two there is another magazine proclaiming another new diet. Of course, they want you to believe that this is the one that will work for you! Just before Christmas of 2021, I saw a magazine that claimed "Drop 45 lbs by Christmas." The date was December 13th. Even if you could do it, that would be totally wrong for your body. You want to avoid those diets at all costs. It isn't healthy to lose weight that quickly and they are precisely the diets that will cause the yoyo effect on your body that we just mentioned. And often you'll be out of pocket because they invariably want to sell you something that in the end doesn't help you much.

So, what am I proposing? Start by eating less food than you are eating now. I know that you've heard all about portion size for perhaps years now. And some of you will claim that you've done it before and it didn't work. I believe you. But if you are serious about losing weight and you have the desire and the will power to do it, then I know that reducing portion size is the place to start. It isn't sexy, and you won't notice results quickly, but it is a starting point. It worked for me and, as I said, I'm just an ordinary person like you, who decided to try this method. My before and after pictures show that it worked and the fact that I've been able to maintain my ideal weight for more than nine years now shows you that it can work for you, too. Combine controlled portion size with some of the other things I do to maintain my weight and you'll see a change, as well. Don't be afraid to follow my suggestions. It really isn't a secret, when you think about it. And it really is the healthiest way to lose weight.

So, what will be the upshot of losing weight in this way? You will become the healthy person that you want to be. You'll look better, you'll feel better, and I know you'll have friends and family who will say to you, "You sure are looking good these days, what is your secret?" And you'll be able to say to them, "There is no secret, really. I've just changed a few things around my diet. I've been able to eat everything I've ever eaten, I've slowly lost weight I didn't need and I've become more fit. I believe that I'm now a happier and healthier person."

It almost always starts with a positive attitude and these folks always approach each day, and life in general, with an attitude that the cup is half full.

a slimmer you

TIPS FROM CHAPTER 2:

1. Have a positive attitude.

2. Look good, feel good.

3. Portion size is a good way to start.

CHAPTER 3
Motivation and Inspiration

In 2009, my wife Bev and I were walking in the woods with our friend Jim Ellis and his wife Linda and he happened to snap the following picture of me. When he sent me this picture, my first reaction was that I looked pregnant. What man wants to think that he looks pregnant? But it was a year before I even considered doing anything about it. When scanning through a number of pictures in July 2010, I discovered this shot again and decided that I had to do something about this look. So, this book is all about what I did and how it worked for me. The following chapters capture the story, but for now I want to say that my journey was slow, methodical, and involved just a few changes in my lifestyle. They weren't big changes but when you add them all together, they worked for me and I learned a lot about myself and how to control my weight. The will power and resolve to stick with my plan of slowly developing a better and healthier body carried me through to my final natural body weight. It wasn't easy at first, but over time it worked. And when you read this book, maybe you'll decide that it can also work for you.

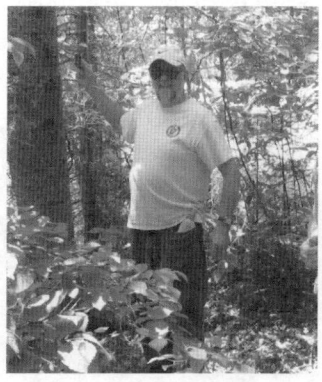

Picture taken in 2009

And that's my intent. To help guide folks to look and feel better about themselves. The final reward is that people stay healthier longer. As I celebrate my success, I hope to celebrate the success of many readers out there like you, who will come to understand that what I'm saying makes sense.

Like many of you, as I was getting on in years. I found it more difficult to accomplish the tasks that were before me. It's not that I couldn't do them, it was just that the extra weight I was carrying made simple chores and duties more difficult. I found that often I was out of breath whenever I hurried to get from one place to another or when I would simply walk up a short flight of stairs. And of course, like so many of us do, I just blamed all my problems on getting older. We are conditioned over our lifetimes to assume that when we age, we will slow down and we won't be able to do what we used to be able to do. And that prophecy does come true if we accept its premise. But what if we were to say no to that stereotype and decide to buck the trend? Then maybe, just maybe, we could pull ourselves up a bit. And what if it were to start by simply losing a little weight and setting a goal of becoming a little more fit? When it works, over time it's like magic. But as you know, weight loss isn't magic and there really are no fast cures.

I know from experience that when you get down to your natural body weight, people you know will mention that you look great. (Especially if they haven't seen you for a while.) They'll say you look younger and guess how that will make you feel? That's right, all of a sudden, you'll walk taller, will seem to have gained renewed confidence, and will feel happier and be proud of your accomplishments.

There will be more about my harvest activities throughout this book but what I want to mention here is that when I got through the 2020 and 2021 harvests, I felt very good. My knees were not bothering me, despite being in and out of tractors, grain trucks, and/or combines over 500 times. Not too bad for an old guy. And I'm out in the fields because I love being out there. But I know there are fellows my age who would love to be out there at harvest but can only sit in their trucks at the edge of the field and watch. Why? Because they're carrying too much weight and their bodies just won't allow them to take an active part in the harvest—something they'd love to be doing. If you are in that category and you have the passion to be contributing at harvest, you can turn it around starting today.

Years ago, my family watched the program "Front Page Challenge" on CBC TV in Canada. If you are my age, and from Canada, you'll recognize the program. It was a weekly program that had "newsmaker guests" come on with three and at times four panelists who had to guess the (mostly hidden) guest's identity by asking questions about what had put them in the headlines. There were strict rules as to what could or couldn't be asked. It really was a show about current events and history. And it was popular in its day, running from 1957 to 1995. That's thirty-eight years on air, covering many guests from several walks of life, including politicians, sports figures, and anyone in between. The only criteria were that they had to have made headlines, either recently or from years before. It was a fine show and afterward, during a short visitation with the panelists, we learned a lot about the contestants and their lives and the headlines that put them on the show.

a slimmer you

One time I was watching "Front Page Challenge" and "Jackrabbit" Johannsen was the guest. He was a Norwegian who had studied engineering in Germany, moved to Cleveland, Ohio, and then to the province of Quebec. In Quebec, he worked for many years with a large number of young people to develop their interest in cross-country skiing. He organized and taught them how to ski properly. He cut many trails through the bush in the Laurentian Mountain area of Quebec. He ran ski races and was an enthusiast for many, many years. He got his nickname because of his ability to move quickly through the bush on his skis. On "Front Page Challenge," Jackrabbit, who must have been close to 100 at the time, was asked, "To what do you owe your longevity?" His instant reply was, "I push back from the table when I feel that I could still eat more!"

At the time I thought that was a very silly and strange answer, and for the next thirty-five years or so, I never gave it much thought. Not until I looked at that picture of myself in 2010. And all of a sudden, the lightbulb came on and Jackrabbit's saying became an inspiration for me. What if I were to start doing what Mr. Johannsen had said? In other words, limiting the amount of food I was consuming at each meal. And, over time, it worked. And that is the essence of this book.

Jackrabbit Johannsen lived to be 111, so you could say that he had caught the secret for living a full, healthy, and enjoyable life. Besides his pushing back from the table statement, another piece of Jackrabbit's advice to live a long and healthy life was to "Stay busy, get plenty of exercise, and don't drink too much. Then again, don't drink too little."

I couldn't help but feel that if this lifestyle worked so well for Jackrabbit Johannsen, then why wouldn't it work for me? And if it worked for me, why couldn't it ultimately work for you, too? If you choose to follow the path I took to meet my goal, you may achieve success with your own weight-loss program, as well.

Recently, my wife Bev and I met Lloyd, a fellow we see frequently when walking our dog Coco on Cloutier Trail near our home in Winnipeg. He's retired and is around the age of sixty-five. We got talking about health and aging and he made the comment, "if someone could guarantee that I'd be healthy up to the age of eighty, I'd take it right now." So, I said to him, "I have the solution for you."

But Lloyd and his wife Jan do walk every day. They used to walk twice a day. The first time was when they walked slowly with their eighteen-year-old golden retriever Orby and they didn't go far. But Orby finally succumbed to old age so they now go on a long, brisk walk every day. Lloyd used to go to the gym when it was open before Covid. And he golfs whenever he gets a chance. He knows I'm writing this book so I'll make sure he gets a copy and I will tell him that the secret to living to a healthy eighty years old is to keep doing what he is already doing while adding a few ideas from this book. I can easily say that to him because I am healthy and am only five years away from the magic eighty age that he has suggested to me. What I've done and continue to do, of course, is no guarantee of him reaching his healthy eighty, but I'm convinced it certainly can help him or anyone attain that goal.

So, what are the benefits of being motivated to lose weight and getting yourself into better physical shape? Well, we've talked about looking younger. Indeed, I am surprised at the number of people who say to me, "You look great." To most of them, I say, "Thanks, you look good, as well." But to some of them who I know well, I'll say, "Thanks, but I work hard to maintain this look." And invariably they'll reply, "I don't doubt it, and it looks like it's working."

And inside I'm quite pleased with their response, but for some of those folks I want to add, "And if you're willing to listen to what I've done to get here, it could work for you, as well." But mostly I just carry on because the one thing I've learned is the old adage, "You can lead a horse to water but you can't make him drink." People have to be ready to quit smoking, or to stop drinking too much, or to stop eating too much. Or to lose weight and get in good physical shape. When people really decide that is what they want to do, they will get started. Many don't know where to start and I'm hoping this book will inspire folks to start by just doing something. And once again I have to mention that there really is no magic to starting and reaching your goals. The best part is that you can start today.

And when you attain your goals, you'll be healthier, you'll be walking more upright, you'll have a better attitude (the glass will be half full rather than the other way around), you'll look better and, guess what, you'll have more pride in yourself as a person. And reaching that magic eighty age with a lilt in your step and a smile on your face, while carrying around a healthier body, will have all been worth it. Isn't that a worthwhile goal for you?

Also, when you and several others accomplish that goal, we end up with a healthier society in general, one that is less of a burden on our health-care system. It's no more evident than right now as we think about all the experiences from the Covid 19 pandemic. Being unhealthy and immune-compromised are not desirable traits to have when there is a deadly virus lurking about. Healthy bodies have a much better chance of warding off a virus like Covid 19. So, having said that, I believe that more people need to make a conscious effort to eat a little less, to lose weight, to move more, to get more exercise, and to set a goal to achieve a body weight that is most natural for their body size and structure. And please don't think I'm preaching to you. I just feel that what has worked for an ordinary guy like me, I know can work for you as well.

Also, before I leave this chapter, I have to share a personal story with you. Back in the mid 1980s, I decided I had to get stronger. I had been living a rather sedentary life so I decided it was time to do something about it. Without conducting any research or soliciting any advice into what I should do for a muscle-building program, I just starting lifting weights with a barbell that we had in our basement at the time. I must have started too fast with too much weight and it wasn't long before I ended up with a hernia. I had an operation to repair the hernia and, over time, I gained back my original strength in that area of my body. But that was a warning to me and I had paid the price. I want it to be a warning to you, as well.

Start slowly, follow my advice on the slow loss of extra weight, be reasonable about your weight-loss program, consult your doctor about what you plan to start doing, and let them know the steps. But most importantly you can start right now. Begin by eating a bit less, get up and get moving and then start following some of the other advice you'll read in this book. Depending on how much weight you have to lose, it may take a while to realize your goals, but believe me, over time, by following these simple steps, you'll see results. Then you'll start feeling better, you'll look different, and you'll walk around with a brand-new attitude. In the end, I know your body will thank you and you'll reach that eighty or ninety age milestone with a healthier body. There'll be only one negative in all this, which will turn into a positive. You'll have to shell out for new clothes (the negative) for your slimmer waistline but you'll look more modern than you have for a while as you walk around proudly in your new duds (the positive). Good luck!

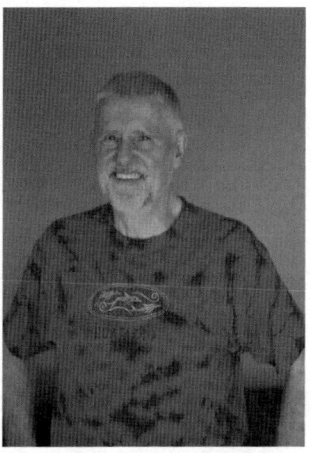

Picture taken in 2022

"I push back from the table when I feel that I could still eat more!"

TIPS FOR CHAPTER 3:

1. Use before pictures for motivation.

2. Strive for a healthy body up to old age.

3. Consult your doctor with your plans.

CHAPTER 4
Eat Less

This is the chapter where you finally learn about how much weight I actually lost and how I managed to lose it. As I've already stated, weight loss isn't magic and can't be accomplished with a snap of the fingers. I believe that if you're serious about losing weight, you must be motivated, you must have a certain level of resolve, and you have to be prepared to stick with your plan. Remember, I didn't set out to lose a lot of weight. When I started, I didn't have a particular goal in mind except that I wanted to lose some weight and no longer look like a pregnant man. Looking ahead, my goal was to have a sideways picture taken of me where I didn't sport that look. So, I told myself, "If I was to actually lose some weight and start looking slimmer, I would have to work diligently at methods and routines that would work for me."

You know that I had already determined that I didn't want to partake in any of the hundreds of diets and programs that were available. I just didn't like the idea of sticking to a program that might help me lose weight and then possibly put the weight right back on. I'd seen that picture with a number of other folks before. And I certainly didn't want to pay for some method of weight loss when I felt I could just start by reducing my overall food intake. I wasn't searching for a drastic weight reduction, just a way of reducing slowly to allow me to shed a few pounds. When I hopped on the scale in July of 2010, I weighed 185 pounds. That was the highest I'd ever weighed in my life and the picture convinced me to do something about it. So, I started by eating less and it worked for the first month. But then I went to my daughter Michelle's wedding in Toronto and, when I got back home, I discovered that the weight I'd lost had come back. Getting those lost pounds back became the catalyst to get serious. I'd just proven to myself that I could actually lose weight. Now I had to learn to lose it and keep it off.

Once I got back on track to losing weight, I shed five pounds over the next few months and thought to myself: *Good. That wasn't easy, but it really wasn't so hard either.* Reducing my food intake started my downward trend. Loading food onto smaller plates also helped. In further chapters you'll read about other changes that helped out, as well. But for now, I was happy to keep losing weight. Over a period of time, maybe a year and a half or so (while experiencing many ups and downs), I was able to get down to 170 pounds. Was I ever proud of myself!

Yes, I'd managed to drop fifteen pounds of weight I didn't need. My waist size was smaller, so that meant a few new pairs of pants. I had to make new holes in my perfectly good belts. Life was rosy. Rosy until I checked what a man of my age and height should weigh. Guess what the answer was? Right there in black and white, the information stated that I should weigh 159 pounds. Wow! I had just worked long and hard to shed fifteen pounds, what I'd done had taken me this far, and now I was supposed to lose eleven more pounds.

After I got over the surprise of learning that I still wasn't near my natural weight, I asked myself, "What now?" But the answer was right before me as you can probably guess. Just keep doing what I'd done to lose the first fifteen and, if successful, then I felt I might reach that suggested goal. At the time, it seemed to be an incredibly far-off goal that I'd never originally set for myself. But maybe, just maybe, it was a goal that could be possible to reach.

So, I continued on with the program that had already worked for me. I ate until I was no longer hungry. (I didn't eat everything that my head told me I really wanted.) I was essentially doing what Jackrabbit Johannsen had promoted so many years before. *I was pushing back from the table when I felt I could still eat more.* But I wasn't eating sparrow meals either, like some folks think they have to, to lose weight. Bev and I believe that in order to have a healthy body, it's necessary to eat three nutritious meals a day and to eat at regular times. When your body knows it'll be fed at a regular time, it seems to expect a meal at that time and I know that you can actually lose weight while eating regularly.

I was now more aware of how eating well and controlling food intake had certainly helped me lose weight over a period of time. I knew it was working. But I had to pause and ask myself if that was enough. When I assessed the regimen that I'd been following, I realized that my reduced food intake, along with other steps, had done the trick to date. And those steps were pushed along by my initial motivation and resolve to shed weight. It actually turned out to be quite a simple way to shed pounds. This whole endeavour helped me lose the extra weight in a most natural way. But was that enough to keep dropping the extra weight? I decided that really, that wasn't enough.

Continuing to go to exercise class, curling twice a week in winter, riding the bike in summer, cross-country skiing in the winter, using urban poles, and walking the dog twice a day all helped with my weight-loss program. There'll be more about that in the chapter on fitness, but I just want to point out here that there are things you can do to assist your weight-loss program. Adopting some or all of these types of things will definitely help. But just in case you think I'm a fitness fanatic, well, guess what? I'm not! Curling twice a week is real, once you sign up you go or you let your team down. Riding the bike is optional, so over a summer I might only ride it ten or twenty times. Not every day like some people I know. Cross-country skiing is optional, so I don't go out in the winter as often as I could or should. Swimming can be done all year round. We have urban poles that we don't use very often but they also help. I guess what I am trying to say here is that anything you do helps. So, if you decide to get up off the couch and start walking, then you'll have accomplished a lot. Combined with less food intake, you will have begun a program for yourself that will start you toward your goals.

I became committed to losing the final eleven pounds. I knew it wouldn't be easy because, as most people have learned, it's the last few pounds of any weight-loss program that are the hardest to get rid of. But I continued along the path that I'd chosen. Maybe I worked a little harder at it. Sweeping harder at curling, being a little more conscious of what was going on my plate, monitoring my weight on the scale, walking a little farther when I was out, pushing my limits on the bicycle, all contributed to help me to shed those last hard-to-get-rid-of pounds.

No matter what you decide for your own program, it's important to remember that it takes a lifetime for a person to reach their maximum weight. We don't wake up one morning to discover that, "poof" the extra pounds **are** there. They just keep creeping up on the body and we don't seem to notice. And the worst of it is, it's like we haven't been paying attention. I'm positive that many of you reading these words will say, "You know, that's right, I never really did pay much attention to what was happening with my body. It's like my body and the scales were playing some kind of a trick on me."

But, remember if you decide to use some of the methods I've used, don't look for instant results. What's important is not that you lose a lot of weight quickly but that the trend starts moving in the right direction. If you lose a few pounds (only to gain them back), it's important to keep in mind exactly what helped you lose those first few pounds. Then go back to it, whatever that was, and get it working for you again. It's said that *patience is a virtue* and, in this case, it truly is. If you want to lose weight fast, then adopt one of those "lose-weight-fast" diets. I don't believe it's healthy to lose weight that way, but they will work for a while. But I'd be surprised if I talked to you a year later and you could honestly say, "I lost fifty pounds in three months and I've kept it off." I would call someone who was successful in doing that an outlier. Why? Because most people I know who have lost weight quickly have gained it all back, and more.

I know I sound like a broken record, but losing weight *slowly* is highly recommended. You do want the downward movement to be slow and steady. Try it for a year and see if your waist size doesn't change in that period of time. But you need to have a strong desire to lose weight and the resolve to accomplish your goals. And as I've said before, if it can work for little ole me, I know it can work for you too.

What helped me to continue on my journey were the several compliments I was getting along the way. Every time I tightened my belt, someone seemed to notice. My daughters all kept telling me they were proud of what I'd accomplished. Close friends also mentioned that I was looking good. Now, to be told that from those closest to you is a very good feeling. It means that you're on the right track to looking good and feeling good. To me, it was a nice reward for having started losing weight and for keeping it off, and it certainly was an incentive to continue to target my natural body weight.

And guess what? My ideal weight did not end up being 159 pounds, it turned out to be 158. This is the weight I got down to and I've been able to keep off the unwanted pounds for nine years now. How come I ended up losing that extra pound? Well, first of all, the determination of what a person of a certain age and height should weigh is not an exact science. Everyone's body is different and the results will vary, of course. But for me, I am very happy to weigh in at 158 pounds. It's a nice even number and the twenty-seven pounds I've lost (and managed to keep off) represent 14.5 percent of body weight (extra fat) that I didn't need. You can do the math for your own body and calculate how many pounds you would get rid of, if that percentage of weight loss also turned out to be your ideal weight. For some, it may be too much but for others it may need to be a higher percentage, but each individual needs to work out what they need to lose. If it's more, it may take longer. But you need to be patient.

In order to maintain my body weight at 158 pounds, I have made a few simple changes to what I was already doing. For instance, I came to realize that, just because food is on the plate, doesn't mean I have to eat it all. We never throw food out as that is not only wasteful but it hits the pocketbook, as well. So often at a restaurant we'll take a doggy-bag home. And the leftover food is definitely not for the dog. She gets her own delicious meals supplemented with scraps from our table. We eat the contents from that doggy-bag in the next day or two. There is no shame in doing so.

Sometimes at home I end up cutting off a third of a delicious hamburger I'm eating. That'll be wrapped to go in the fridge for a snack at another time. Same with a super tasty medium rare steak. I like to prepare and barbecue steaks to a savoury, mouth-watering level of doneness. But I only take what I need for that particular meal. The next day, the rest of the steak will be cut into little chunks to be lightly fried and served as steak and eggs (only one egg, though) for breakfast or the leftover steak will be shaved and added to a salad for lunch. Nothing is wasted and delicious meals are always created and enjoyed as leftovers. It's good to be creative and it continues to be important not to eat more than your body needs. In other words, *push back from the table when you feel you could still eat more!*

Anything you do can help, so if you decide to get up off the couch and start walking, then you'll have accomplished a lot.

TIPS FROM CHAPTER 4:

1. Set your weight-loss goal and stick with it.

2. Fitness classes will help.

3. Start moving now and into the future.

CHAPTER 5
The Goal

So, this is the meat of my story on weight loss. It's really a story of getting started and working with determination, resolve, and a certain degree of will power. We all know that the key to weight loss is nothing more than burning more calories that we consume in a given day. But is it actually that simple? If that's true and we've been trying for years to lose weight, why hasn't it worked?

I've mentioned this before but there have been hundreds of diets advertised throughout my lifetime, and recently there are many new ones promising instant results over a short period of time. I won't name any of them, but you know what these diets are. They scream out at you from the magazine counters as you head to the checkout at your grocery store. Maybe you've tried some of those diets only to gain the weight back again.

For a time, those diets do work, because it's like New Year's resolutions, many folks *want* to lose weight so they tell themselves on January 1st every year, "*This is the ye*ar." And they start with great intentions and, for a while, it works. Gyms have an influx of new clients every January and, often, by the end of the month, attendance starts to drop off. People retain their memberships but don't regularly attend. It's the same with many diets that claim unbelievable weight-loss numbers. Yes, they may help a few folks on a continuous basis, but for many others, the early successes come to a rapid end. And the consequence is that the pounds that were lost come back—and sometimes more are added.

So, what can you do? Well, as you know, there is no silver bullet to weight loss, but the easiest first step is to simply start to eat less. And it really is a lot easier than you might think. We aren't as active as we once were and of course our age is a big factor. When I think of all the grain I shovelled or bales I had to pick up and carry, or pails of water or feed I hauled to the turkeys, I realize that I was a heck of a lot more active than I am now. So back in those days I could eat as much as I wanted, whenever I wanted. I was burning calories off big time.

Professional and Olympic athletes burn a lot of calories and of course they need to consume more food in order to keep their bodies in top competitive shape. But most of us just don't fit that category and the more we sit around, the more we add and keep extra pounds that our bodies don't need.

It's well known that, to maintain a healthy body and a steady weight, most adults (especially those of us at a certain age) should eat the equivalent of 2,000 calories a day. Some days it will be higher and other days it might be lower but it needs to stay close to 2,000. And, of course you'll need to burn off some of those calories but we'll talk more about that later. Not long ago I read that the average American eats around 3,770 calories a day. Where do you suppose those extra 1770 calories are going? That's right, they're stored as fat in the body. Weight goes up and waistlines increase. And lest we get smug about our own eating habits, statistics show that the average Canadian eats 3419 calories per day.

However, you know the obvious, that everyone is different in body size and height. So, consider the results of a 2004 government overview of Canadian eating habits. It states that a thirty-year-old man who is five feet nine inches tall and weighs 165 pounds needs 2750 calories a day, whereas a sedentary sixty-five-year-old woman who is 5 feet 1 inch tall and weighs 132 pounds needs 1,600 calories a day. But, an active twelve-year-old boy who is four feet eleven inches tall and weighs around 100 pounds needs 2,625 calories a day. Consequently, it's easy to see that everyone's needs are different. And of course, the less active you are, the fewer calories you should be consuming to maintain your body weight.

I want you to know one sure-fire method to start on a journey to losing weight. For me it was to start using smaller plates. The average dinner plate in our kitchen is ten-and-three-quarter inches in diameter but the next size down is a luncheon plate which is nine inches across. At home, we started to back away from dinner plates to serve our meals and went to the nine-inch plate. Can you guess the percent difference in area between the two plates? If you were in one of my seminars, I would get you to write down your guess and the closest to the right answer would get a small prize. But I will tell you now that the difference in area between the two plates is close to 42.5 percent. And I've seen people at a buffet that I've mentioned before, load a big plate up right to the edge and then go back for another helping of at least two-thirds of that plate size again. They are consuming at least 50 percent or more than if they loaded up a nine-inch plate once. Where are the extra calories going that they're consuming every day? That's right, stored in the body as fat, mainly in the gut area.

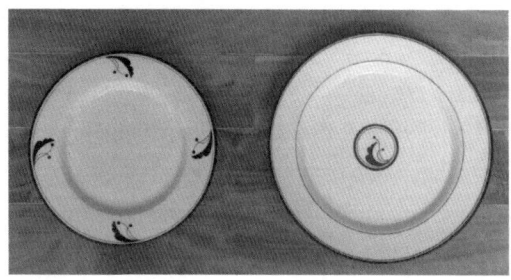

The difference in area size between dinner vs. luncheon plates is 42.5 percent

a slimmer you

I want to share a story about a study I heard of on the radio. It was a test to see if people helping themselves at a buffet actually believed they needed as much food as they were taking. Diners were allowed to go through the buffet and fill up their plates with all the food they wanted. (Or that they thought they wanted.) At first the only plates available to them were the bigger dinner plates. Those conducting the experiment waited for folks to go through and load their plates with food as they normally would. But when the diners got to the end of the line, the experimenters said, "We're very sorry for the inconvenience, but we understand that the plates you have in your hands were not properly cleaned and we don't want anyone to get sick. If you will kindly give us your plate, we'll replace it with a clean plate and you'll be able to go through the line again."

Everyone who co-operated was then given a luncheon plate and they went through the buffet again. This time when the participants loaded up again, they of course could not take as much as the first time because of the smaller plate size. When the experiment was over, the researchers determined that most people in the study ended up eating just two-thirds of what they had initially taken. The diners reported that they were full and did not go back for more food to make up for what had initially been taken away. It sort of says that in an affluent society like ours, we tend to eat more food than our bodies need. Especially if we're living a sedentary lifestyle.

So really, the above experiment was an exercise of controlling portion size. But I've heard people say, "Portion size, portion size. If I hear one more word about portion size, I'm going to throw my plate at the wall." Therefore, I'll refrain from using the term too much in this book but I do want to tell you that going to smaller plate sizes and sticking to it was what helped me on my weight-loss journey. Getting down to my natural weight over three years began with eating less from smaller plates continues to this day. There's a story coming up soon where we went away from the smaller plate size practice and ended up paying a small price.

I really want you to understand that the reason I am so committed to the cause of eating less to lose weight is because I did not have to give up anything. That's right. I enjoy my food just like most people. I like to experience the five tastes that are offered by the various foods we eat. As a refresher they are sweet, sour, salty, bitter and umami. We are all familiar with the first four and we know what foods provide those tastes. But some folks may not know what umami is and how it fits in as a taste. Umami comes from the Japanese culture and is described as "the essence of deliciousness." It provides a meaty savory taste in the mouth and is found in foods like mushrooms and avocados. Umami helps to heighten the flavours of the other four tastes. If you're unfamiliar with it as a taste, check the internet for more information about it.

My wife Bev is a foodie (person who loves to cook with good, fresh ingredients and enjoys creating kitchen masterpieces) who loves to please me with new as well as my favourite tried-and-true recipes. We have some type of dessert (which may be fruit) after every lunch and dinner. My chosen way of losing weight and keeping the pounds off allows me to enjoy everything I've ever eaten in my life—foods that include all meats (especially steak), vegetables (corn is my favourite), pulses, bread, pasta, pizza, ice cream, cakes, muffins, pies, and every other type of food I have enjoyed all my life. In plain language, I never quit eating anything that I like or have a desire to eat. So, what is the secret?

I just started to take in less food and that meant leaving behind extra calories I didn't need. I no longer eat bread or buns with my meals. Slowly but surely, my weight began to go down. I have to say that once I started to use smaller plates, my weight-loss journey turned out to be less difficult than you might think. Once I started the downward trend and became pleased about what I was seeing on the scale, it all just seemed to fit into place like a puzzle. And I should remind you once again that I never started with the idea of losing a lot of weight. My idea at the beginning was to just lose a few pounds and *not* look pregnant.

It's been said that the first bite and the last bite are the only ones that count. In other words, the first bite of a piece of chocolate cake, for instance, is the best and most wonderful taste you have of the beautiful cake you've been eyeing up. It looks delicious and you know it is. So, you're excited for the first bite and it lives up to its expectations. Wow! Then as you eat through the piece of cake the initial desire starts to relax and the last bite is the one that determines when you might want another piece of that chocolate cake. What I'm saying here is that after a big meal, when you tie into that chocolate cake, if you eat too big a piece, the last bite will not leave you wanting more for a while. A smaller piece might mean you'll want to eat chocolate cake sooner and you go through the savouring routine all over again. Hopefully this helps you understand the importance of the first and last bite.

What I've found by reducing my food intake is that when it comes to desserts, I enjoy them over a longer period of time. I used to eat a full-on piece of pie or cake or whatever was the dessert of the day. Then I might have another half piece because the first one tasted so good. But guess what? The pie or cake didn't last very long. Now I take one smaller piece each time and even though I want more, I just resist the urge. So that pie that lasted only two or three days before, might now last up to five days and I get to enjoy its delicious taste over several days. And I like experiencing that. Each day brings the same desires and thoughts as the first day did.

And here is another little trick I learned. At a buffet where there are a number of desserts, I usually want to try more than one because they all look delicious. But I can't possibly eat two or three of the size that have been cut. I carry a small knife on my belt and I'll just cut the desserts in half and I get to enjoy several small bites of a number of them. Do I worry about getting in trouble? Not at all. I've never been told not to do that. And besides, I can guarantee you that behind me is someone who says, "Look at that half-sized piece of pie or cake. It's just the amount I want." That happens all the time and I know from having done it that when I go back a short time later (or even before I leave the buffet line), that dessert I had cut in half and left behind is gone. Just like magic!

The point of all this is that just because you decide to lose weight doesn't mean you have to give up any of the foods you love and enjoy. Try eating less of all your favourite foods and your enjoyment of them continues while you lose the extra pounds you don't need.

When I decided to lose weight, I made up my mind to go easy at the table so I started by only cooking one egg at breakfast. We don't always have sausages or bacon, but when we do, I now cook only two breakfast sausages instead of four or five, or one strip of bacon rather than three or four. And I'll limit the number of slices of toast to two, always with our homemade jam or peanut butter and honey. For lunch and supper with small plates, I will cut back on everything, just like at breakfast.

At buffets, because it is so easy to get side-tracked, I consciously started taking less food. If it was at breakfast, I learned to take fewer sausages or strips of bacon and I'd take a small scoop of scrambled eggs not three like I used to. And again, two pieces of toast is enough. If it were a lunch or dinner buffet, I learned to take two to three meatballs and small slab of meat off the roast or ham that was offered, not four to six meatballs and a large slab or two off the roast. A small number of potatoes and veggies or salad is now the norm versus the all-you-can-eat version like in the past. If perogies are offered, I take two to three of them, not four to six, like I used to. Moderation is the key. I always try to keep in mind the 2,000 calories a day that my body needs.

When you learn to eat smaller amounts of food this way, then it's a snap to leave the table after a satisfying meal and get down on the floor to play with grandchildren or even join them in a rousing game of soccer or floor hockey or other game. I no longer feel that I need a rest after meals, which I often did after consuming more food than I needed.

I want to finish this chapter with a true story that happened in pre-covid days. My oldest daughter Laura had created a very delicious turkey dinner with all the fixings. She brought out her best dinner plates, which of course are bigger than what my wife Bev and I are used to filling up. Guess what? Both of us mistakenly filled our bigger plates with delicious food and proceeded to eat it all, followed by dessert. By the time we got home, both of us admitted to each other that we were feeling uncomfortable because of the extra food we'd eaten but didn't need. So beware, if you get used to eating smaller portions served on smaller plates, you have to remember that when you're given a bigger plate, try to avoid loading it up. Your stomach will remind you later that it wasn't the smartest idea you had that day.

Getting down to my natural weight over three years began with smaller plates and continues to this day.

TIPS FROM CHAPTER 5:

1. Use smaller plates.

2. Our bodies need 2,000 calories/day.

3. When you control food intake, you'll shed pounds.

CHAPTER 6
Fad Diets Don't Work

We've all seen the ads advocating for immediate results with popular weight-loss diets. They're everywhere. They promise the moon of losing twenty to thirty pounds or more in a very short time. They are enticing and many folks buy in to this advertising but in the end, many of these diets fail. Sure, people almost always lose weight because that's the main goal, but it isn't long before the unwanted pounds reappear. Why does that happen over and over again? It's because our bodies aren't geared to lose weight fast. Heck, just think about the amount of time it took you to get to your present weight. It may have taken several years to put on those extra pounds. So, if it took that long to put it on, doesn't it make sense that those pounds should be shed in a slow and methodical manner? I'm a good advocate of slow weight-loss, because it absolutely worked for me and I believe it can work for you as well.

Every one of us knows people who have been on yoyo diets. Did they work? Yes, for a time, but for the most part, the person gained the weight back. And some folks have tried more than one of these diets. Each diet promised a slim, trim body in a matter of weeks or months. Often, there are testimonials and pictures of people who have successfully lost weight. But we may not see pictures of those same people six months or a year or two later. You never will, because promoters of these diets want money that folks are willing to fork over to pay for their programs or their particular brand of supplements. Or it might be the promotion of a protein mix that you absolutely need to sustain a healthy body. But what is wrong with getting what your body needs from the foods that you eat?

So, what is the definition of a fad diet? Simply stated, it's a diet that promises quick weight loss but ultimately is unhealthy because it doesn't provide required nutrition. These diets aren't at all like a diet that is varied with a number of different wholesome and nutritious foods. A diet that regularly includes fresh fruits, fresh vegetables, wholesome meats or fish—in other words, food that you've prepared yourself so you know exactly what you are consuming.

From the internet, I was able to learn that fad diets do indeed lead to weight loss, but they just aren't a healthy choice. What people lose immediately is water weight, not the fat that has caused the weight problems in the first place. So, initially folks believe that the fad diet is working. Often the intake of healthy foods is limited and people end up eating foods with less nutrition and fewer calories. The body might be deprived of the nutrients it needs and problems can occur, such as headaches, weakness, nausea, dehydration, and constipation.

"The best approach for losing weight is to eat a healthy diet and to do regular exercises," claims one site where I checked for information on this topic. And another claims that fad diets are for those people who want to burn off calories without doing any physical activities. If people are tired of being overweight, fad diets are not the answer. There are a number of problems with fad diets, particularly when a person stays on them for too long. At the extreme end, people can lose hair, their nails can become brittle, their skin can lose its shine, and dark circles can appear under the eyes. That's because the essential vitamins, minerals, and nutrients that are required for proper bodily functions are often missing. The whole scenario points to an unhealthy choice.

The April 20, 2021, issue of *Reader's Digest* covers off the topic of four reasons why fad diets are bad for you:

1. *You end up feeling dehydrated:* When you lose weight too fast, the quick weight loss is due to water loss from the body. If you try to force your body to lose weight faster than it naturally wants to, you can end up with serious health problems. So, a recommendation to avoid overeating is to drink one or two glasses of water before a meal. And if you exercise daily, drink more water to replace the water lost from sweating.

2. *You get tired quickly:* Fad diets deprive the body of calories that provide energy to help you get through the day. If you fast or eat less than what your body requires in order to lose weight too quickly, you'll find yourself feeling fatigued for most of the day. As a counter-balance, eat smaller meals throughout the day. This helps boost your metabolism and can provide more energy to help you lose weight in a healthy manner.

3. *You can get serious digestive problems:* Losing weight too quickly can lead to severe diarrhea over an extended period of time which can lead to dehydration—and that can be life threatening. And one recommendation to counteract that problem is to make sure to get an adequate amount of fibre in your diet.

4. *You'll suffer from malnutrition:* Crash diets and fasting are dangerous because they restrict you from consuming fats and carbs, and they're also unsafe since they prevent your body from getting the vitamins and minerals it needs. If you restrict your body from its normal caloric intake over a long period of time, your body will be deprived of its essential nutrients and you'll become severely malnourished. A major tip is that a healthy, well-balanced diet is the key to proper weight loss.

And that's the main theme for this book and especially for this chapter. If you want to lose weight in a healthy way, keep eating what your body is already used to, just start by eating a little less at each meal. And make sure to consult with your health-care professional (doctor, nurse practitioner, etc.) to make sure that what you are doing is right for you and your body. I'm sure they will have a number of guidelines for you to follow. And just remember folks, *if it sounds too good to be true, then it probably is.*

When I started on my weight-loss journey, I lost four pounds in the first month and gained it back when I went to my daughter's wedding in Toronto. When I got back, I had to start over and this time I promised myself I would stick with the program and try to reach my weight loss goal. That goal was just to lose a few pounds, to keep it off and to look better. That was twelve years ago now. Little did I know at the time that the whole experience would lead to the book you are now reading. Slowly over 3 years I reached what I now consider is the ideal weight for me. (158 pounds) And I'm totally convinced that this is the only way to lose weight in a healthy manner. And as you can see, it has worked. Not only did I lose extra weight I didn't need, I've kept it off successfully for the last nine years and counting.

Remember when I referred to the picture that my friend Jim Ellis took of me and I didn't like the profile. Well, when I told him that was what started me on my weight-loss journey, Jim said, "If I'd known it was going to have that kind of an impact on you, then I wouldn't have taken that picture." And my answer to that is, "no, no, no!" If I hadn't seen that picture, then I might not have started on my journey to lose weight. It definitely was my motivation to start losing weight and to keep it off. Without getting kick-started like that, I wouldn't be able to play with my grandchildren so easily as I do, or work in the fields during harvest (a true passion) or run races at the Manitoba fifty-five-plus games. I would have been too heavy to do those things and I believe my knees would have given out from the burden of supporting the extra weight.

Having said that, I want you to consider what an English registered dietician, Sue Baic who is a spokesperson for the British Dietetic Association has said about losing weight and what it means to the knee joint. Sue says, *"For every 0.5 kg (or 1 pound) of weight lost, we reduce the weight going through the knee joint at each step by 2 kg (or 4.5 pounds)."* That fact might not mean much until you put some real figures behind it. I lost twenty-seven pounds during my weight loss program. That means I've reduced the pressure on my knees by the equivalent of a whopping *one hundred and twenty-one and a half* pounds with each step I take. Once I absorbed and understood that information, I was so happy to realize that over the last decade I was able to protect my knees from that extra punishment. And it certainly is food for thought for those people who have been fighting weight their whole life. It's no wonder that you see so many older folks walking with a limp from bad knees or bad hips. There's been a lot of extra pressure on those joints for so many years. If you choose to do something about it now, it can certainly pay off in the future.

I'll mention this again in Chapter 16, but for many farmers who enjoyed being around equipment and being in the fields all their lives, it's tough to be a half-ton observer. There are a number of folks who can no longer climb up into a tractor to operate a grain cart, or climb into a combine or withstand the rigours of climbing in and out of a truck to haul grain. And they find it impossible to put in a long day in the field. Their joints and back just would not hold up long enough for them to get through a harvest season. Even though the machines are so much easier to operate, that really doesn't come into play if the poor old body doesn't want to co-operate.

So, I want to throw out a caution flag to all you thirty-five, fifty, and sixty-year-old folks out there who would like to still be an active part of the farming operation when you're in your seventies and eighties. If you're starting to get a bit paunchy and have to buy a bigger belt to accommodate your expanding waistline, then think about reversing that process. Start losing weight now, work at getting and staying fit and you'll be doing your knee and hip joints a big favour. Then you'll be able to be a part of the family farming operation for a longer time than you might otherwise. I'm an example of someone who has accomplished that goal and I'm so happy to have done it. I'm sure that you would be as well.

But my advice isn't just for farmers. That's a group I've been closest to all my life and they are near and dear to my heart. This advice is for anyone who has been participating in activities they've enjoyed all their lives. Be it water-skiing, downhill skiing, cross-country skiing, swimming, playing tennis, squash, racquetball, basketball, baseball, hockey or golf. You'll be able to perform any one of those sports much later in your life if you decide to shed some extra pounds now, pounds that your body doesn't need. This is not a condemnation of your current life-style by any means, I just want you to know that if you plan for a healthier future now, then your body will be able to cope better in that future. And you'll be in better shape to handle any health set-backs that might occur. Isn't that a reasonable goal to aim for?

I'm hoping that what I've written so far makes sense to you the reader. And if you need more confirmation about the overall benefits of a healthy body and a healthy mind just keep reading. There is lots of information to absorb but I believe it's very relevant to anyone who wants to look into their crystal ball and see themselves as they imagine how they'd like to look when they're in their seventies and eighties or older. There are many examples and role models out there to pattern your life after. You see a number of folks struggling with walkers and canes and some in wheelchairs as a result of bad knees, hips or as a result of a stroke or a premature heart attack. Much of it caused from simply carrying more weight for too many years when they were younger.

Or, you can model yourself after a person like Jackrabbit Johannsen who was forever fit, and who pushed back from the table when he felt he could still eat more. And remember, he lived a healthy life until he was 111. You have to decide for yourself what lifestyle is best for you. There are choices you can make for yourself. Take a little time to think about it and I'm hoping you'll make the choice that will benefit you in the healthiest way for your body and for your future. Just go for it!! I know you can do it!

A fad diet is a diet that promises quick weight loss but ultimately is one that is unhealthy and is often unbalanced.

TIPS FOR CHAPTER 6:

1. Avoid fad diets.

2. Eat healthy, well-balanced meals.

3. Losing excess weight benefits the joints.

CHAPTER 7
The Scales

Another key part of my weight-loss program has been the bathroom scale. I think it cost me under ten dollars and it has been worth every single penny and more. Why? Because I use it to monitor my daily progress. For many of us (like I used to do), if we weigh once in a while it seems to be enough. However, when a person only weighs infrequently, then often you hear comments like, "the scales must be lying, or where did that come from?" The realization that you've eaten too much, snacked too much or not exercised enough is always revealed through your scale. Big surprise folks, there's nothing wrong with your scale.

I know people who say they wouldn't own a scale because it always shows they are overweight. Well, guess what, I believe owning a scale is very important and using it regularly is an important habit to get into. Why? It's because the scale constantly monitors the trend of what is happening to my body weight. Without consciously being aware, unwanted weight sneaks up and the next thing I know, I might be ten to twelve pounds heavier than I want or need to be. Daily weighing allows me to monitor if I'm going up in weight, staying the same or dropping down a bit. Dropping is good but somehow, I always gain those pounds back. When I notice my weight going the wrong way (i.e., I'm getting heavier) then I adjust my eating and or fitness habits slightly to get back on track. Without constantly being aware of my body weight, all of a sudden, I might weigh more than I want to. It's very easy for unwanted pounds to accumulate. So, my advice to you when you decide to start your weight-loss program, is to use your scale to monitor your incremental steps downwards. Little triumphs like two pounds lost over ten days or two weeks is monumental in the scheme of things. But without weighing every day, how would you know if those two pounds are gone? It's so important to be aware of your weight trend downwards. The scale is your management tool that keeps you focused. And besides, the sooner you start using it to monitor your progress, the easier it gets. You start off in the morning with no clothes on, so remembering to weigh yourself before putting them on or before showering becomes routine.

Since I've shed those unneeded pounds, I've itemized newly gained weight into two separate categories that I call soft pounds and hard pounds. Soft pounds are those that I might add when I eat differently from my daily routine. Perhaps it's because I've had the occasion to dine out more times than usual. Often circumstances happen that way. Perhaps, I've been to dinner with friends and they've prepared a gorgeous meal complete with a scrumptious dessert. How could I resist? Anyway, after that kind of week, because of weighing every day I realize I'm up two to three pounds. See, I've noticed the trend and have to adjust accordingly. It may take up to five days to lose that weight but I know it's important to get rid of them and I make it happen. Reduced food intake and a more rigorous ride on my bike or on the skis for a day or two will usually help me back up again. Because it doesn't take long to get back to my natural weight, I call these *soft* pounds.

Now to the hard pounds. Those are extra pounds that a person might put on during an extended time of celebration such as at Christmas. It's all there. Most cooks like to perform their best around the festive season. Almost all of us love the turkey, stuffing, cranberry sauce, gravy, mashed potatoes, turnips, peas, corn, other veggies, dressings, salads, special breads, and mouth-watering desserts like pies and cakes and ice cream. You name it! The sky is the limit. And of course, there seems to be limitless bowls of candy, mandarin oranges, chocolates, chips, pretzels and fudge. Makes the mouth water just listing it all. And we can't forget the leftovers the next day and beyond. Don't we love to fill up a big bun with lots of turkey, dressing, gravy, cranberry sauce and other favourite fixings, and fill another plate of everything we had the previous day including desserts? Some folks have plum pudding covered in the special brown-sugar sauce. Mmm, delicious.

This type of eating may go on for a few days with not much movement away from the house because for many Canadians it's the week to watch the exciting annual World Junior Hockey tournament. And during that time drinks and snacks have to be tied to the annual ritual. Then New Year's Eve comes along which involves more eating and drinking. Why not? It's what people do when they celebrate the festive season.

Years ago, I read that the average North American (who celebrates Christmas) will gain 8 pounds during the festive season. I believe it and for some folks it will be even more. Gyms and other exercise outlets benefit from Christmas over-indulgences. New Year's Resolutions abound.

These added pounds gained over the holiday season are what I call *hard* pounds. Why? Because there are so many of them, they are harder to get rid of. They are the same hard pounds that a person might accumulate on a ten-to-fourteen-day cruise. I've heard about the delicious buffets and dining rooms that are open twenty-four-seven aboard those ships. It would be hard for me to avoid visiting those food locations far more often than would be healthy for me. And I can just visualize all the wonderful pies and cakes that are calling out for my dining pleasure. Hard pounds indeed!

Having outlined the difference, you know that with the help of my simple bathroom scale, I've been able to control both soft and hard pounds for over nine years. I've determined that my natural weight is 158 pounds. I know that because whenever I drop a few pounds below 158, it doesn't seem long before I'm back at that weight. If I add two or three extra pounds after eating a few bigger meals or too many sweets or snacks, it doesn't seem too difficult to slip back down to 158. It really is just being aware of what's going on with my body and the scale is my daily buddy. It certainly doesn't lie to me. It might make me angry sometimes but it never lies.

I weigh every morning in the nude. That's right, in the nude. Why? Because after a good night's sleep, in the morning after using the washroom, before showering and before putting anything into my mouth, is when I believe a person's body is at its lowest weight of the day. Your body has had time to metabolize the meal from the day before and there is no weight from water, coffee or your delicious one egg meal and toast. Step on the scale before going to the kitchen and watch what the scale is trying to tell you. When you weigh every day, then you know what will happen when you hop on the scale. If you've eaten normally and exercised to the same degree as you've been doing, you'll basically weigh the same within a few tenths of a pound one way or the other. If you've had an especially big or late evening meal or eaten more snacks than usual, then you know you'll be up in weight when you climb onto the scale. Being body-aware is so important here.

To support my idea of weighing nude, I want to share a story about going to my doctor. For years I'd been going for an annual check-up where a nurse would ask me to step on a scale and record my weight. Well, one time when I was there, I asked if it was okay if I took off my shoes, and was told I could take off whatever I wanted (within reasonable protocols), so I took off my shoes and unloaded my pockets of wallet, keys and coins. I think I even took off my belt. My weight was taken and my doctor asked me if I'd lost ten pounds. Without explaining to him what I'd done before having my weight taken, I said, "No, I've been the same weight for the last six years." He must have been baffled but we carried on. All the extra things on my body weighed ten pounds. I'd never expected that or thought about it before. It's a simple lesson to explain why weighing nude gives you your true body weight every morning.

Now, if you've been using digital scales, you know that sometimes when you stand on them differently than the last time you weighed, you might get a wonky measurement. For instance, without changing your diet or anything else you've been doing recently, the scale might show you to be heavier by four pounds say or lighter by that same amount. Because you've been weighing every day, you automatically know that there is something wrong. So, I advise carefully getting on the scale one more time and you should come up with a more normal reading. But please don't become obsessive about jumping on the scale more than a couple of times. I know people who are so obsessed with their weight that they weigh themselves twelve or more times a day. It's not something that I agree with or advocate anyone doing.

Using the scale is like investing money in a long-range portfolio. You use it to follow the trends of your body weight. It isn't the end-all and be-all. The scale is just another tool for you to use in your weight-loss program. In long-range investments, a financial advisor follows the trends. He or she will advise you not to jump in or out of your investments just because the market swings higher one week or takes a big dip the next week. People lose money by jumping in and out of the markets whenever they detect a change. Staying invested by following the long-term trends is what your financial advisor wants you to do. When you obey the trends over the long haul, then you'll end up with a solid financial portfolio. It's the same with your weight loss program. Once you're committed to it and you use the scale to follow your trends (up or down), you'll be satisfied with your final reward. A natural body weight that's correct for your age and your physical body size.

Hopefully I've convinced you that following your weight trends by weighing every day will benefit you through your weight loss program. Remember if you trend down from your natural body weight, that's not a bad thing. I know from experience that eventually you will put on those pounds again. It does happen and you'll be surprised about how quickly it does. But when it goes the other way and you're adding a few pounds you need to be vigilant. If you are up, say two pounds, it's not that much of a problem, your body can easily handle that. What the scale helps you avoid is gaining a few more pounds over a few weeks and then a few more. Weighing every day shows that this is happening and you need to adjust your habits to get back to your natural weight.

I know that my weight will be up after Thanksgiving and Christmas! I make no apologies for that as these are festive seasons after all and I always plan to "pig-out". (My apologies to any barnyard pigs who might be offended by reading this.) By weighing every day, I discover how bad my eating sins are and over time, I do the combination of eating less and exercising more. Whatever it takes to get back to one hundred and fifty-eight pounds (my natural body weight). I hope you understand why I say the scale is my friend. It helps me to spot the trends and adjust accordingly. This past fall I had dropped five pounds just by being more active over the summer. I wasn't concerned and sure enough, the fresh veggie season hit complete with corn-on-the-cob and over three weeks I had gone up past my natural body weight. Without following what was happening on the scale I wouldn't have known that I was trending up. I had to lower my corn consumption along with the other delicious fresh produce.

Recently, I heard a personal trainer on the radio say that she doesn't recommend that people weigh themselves every day. She claimed that a number of her clients are in the process of changing fat to muscle and they may not see their weight changing and become discouraged. That's fine to suggest that those types of clients not weigh themselves every day. Those aren't the people I address in this book. I want to show ordinary people like you that it's possible to live a healthier lifestyle. Folks who are older and who may be living a sedentary lifestyle, who may not be very active and who may have gained extra weight.

The scale certainly helped me to stay on track as I dropped from 185 to 158 pounds and as I've said it has helped me maintain that weight for nine years and holding. I'll never stop weighing every day.

Trust that the scale will help you spot increases or decreases in your weight, that it will work for you and the next thing you know you might be shedding weight you don't want.

When you recognize the difference between soft and hard pounds and learn not to panic when they appear, you'll be on your way to controlling your own natural body weight. It's a weight that should be comfortable for your body size and shape. You know how hard you have to work to keep shedding extra pounds. But when it all comes together, you'll be *A Slimmer*

a slimmer you

You. You'll have created a healthier body that looks good, feels good and is good. And like me you'll enjoy the compliments of family and friends as well as those from strangers who often won't believe your actual age. In my case, I owe much of my accomplishments to my lowly bathroom scale.

Using the scale is like investing your money in a long-range portfolio. You use it to follow the trends of your body weight.

TIPS FROM CHAPTER 7:

1. The scale is your friend.

2. A key is to control soft and hard pounds.

3. Overeating has to be monitored.

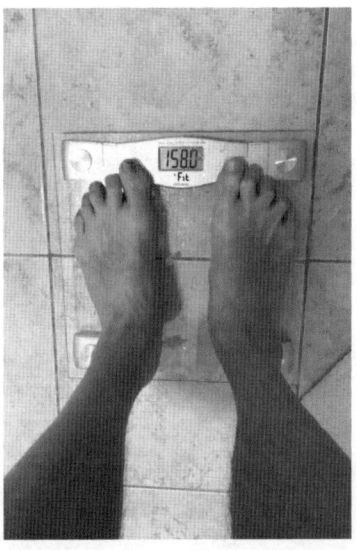

Over the years a steady 158 pounds

CHAPTER 8
Getting Fit

How does losing weight and being fit go hand-in-hand to help create a healthier person? The answer is quite simple. Being fit allows us to do the things we want to do. In the next chapter we'll learn about specific exercises that help us accomplish those goals but for this chapter I asked an acquaintance, Dr. Richard Blouw for some of his observations. Dr. Blouw was a Family Physician for over forty years and served as chairman of the Family Practise Department at Victoria Hospital in Winnipeg for many years. And through most of his career he taught post-graduate students in Family Medicine at the University of Manitoba.

One of the first things Dr. Blouw mentioned was that, "Exercise is not nearly as efficient a means of losing weight compared to the number of calories a person eats, but exercise is a key component to both quality of life and longevity. Low fitness levels are strong predictors of earlier death, much more-so than being overweight alone."

What he writes is that we can lose weight by eating less (the main premise of this book), but getting and staying fit allows us to enjoy life to its fullest. When a person is fit, he or she can accomplish so many more things like travelling, hiking, running long or short distances, walking the dog, gardening, riding a bike, carrying groceries in without discomfort, pushing open heavy doors, skiing (downhill or cross-country), swimming, paddling, kayaking, playing baseball, curling or taking part in age related games like the annual fifty-five-plus games in your respective province. And age need not be a limitation for any of those activities if a person is determined to become fit and remain fit.

Dr. Blouw also adds, "The following are some of the benefits of exercise: reduced levels of diabetes, lower levels of dementia, decreased hip fracture risk, reduced risks of knee or hip replacement surgery, lower levels of arthritis, reduced levels of anxiety and depression, less fatigue, lower blood pressure, a decreased risk of certain cancers, better sleep, lower levels of heart disease, and (above all) an improved quality of life!"

That list outlines many reasons to be fit, by a man who has seen it all over his lifetime practise. Don't his observations make you want to get up and get moving? We all know how easy it is to go everywhere by vehicle. It's not uncommon to see people hop in their car or SUV and travel just a few short blocks. But we know that there are many benefits to hopping on a bike or just plain walking to that same destination. And once a person is fit, as long as they keep doing what they did to get to that level of fitness, it becomes much easier to continue doing it.

I don't want you to think I'm advocating that everyone become a gym rat. We will leave that type of fitness training to high powered athletes (both amateur and professional). Although I often see folks older than myself working out at the gym and they are very fit, I want to address folks who are around my age and who might have been living a sedentary lifestyle. I'm hoping they become determined to get up, shed some pounds in a healthy way, and start a fitness program that is correct for their body size and capability and that they'll start as soon as possible. Baby steps are fine to get started and then it becomes easier to make major strides. Over a short period of time when you've shed some weight and begun to get fit, you'll find that weight loss and fitness actually do complement each other.

When I was seventy, I decided to run in the fifty-five-plus games that have been held in Manitoba since 1983. Although I never ran the 100 metres (100 yards back in my time) before, I decided to give it a try and did a bit of training ahead of time. I didn't know what to expect, but I entered in my age class and ran at the games at Killarney, Manitoba. I surprised myself with a time of 17.79 seconds and was pleased to win a gold medal. (A little secret here, there was no competition in my class but I did run against runners in other classes.) It was a fun thing to do. But the most exciting for me was when a year later at Glenboro, Manitoba, I decided to run the 100 and the 200 metres as well. I did not practise at all for the 200, as I just felt that once a person gets by the 100-metre mark, you just keep running and that was what I did. My time in the 100 metres was slower than the first year but I was very excited about my time in the 200 metres. It was 38.29 seconds. If that doesn't mean much to you, consider this. At the time, I was exactly three times as old as Andre De Grasse, who is Canada's premiere world-class sprinter. His time for the 200 metres that year was 19.95 seconds. If you were to compare our times based on age alone, my time should have been 59.85 seconds. But it was actually less than double his time. De Grasse at the time was a very healthy 24-year-old, who has very strong thighs and who trains every day leading up to major track meets. So, I felt really good about my time in the 200 metres, especially after not even training to run it. Could I have reached that time if I still weighed 185 pounds? Not a chance and I think that will be obvious to anyone reading this.

Also, at the Killarney 55+ games, there was a woman over 80 years old who ran great times in the 100, 200, 400 and 1500 metre races. I asked her if she trained hard for the games and she replied, "I don't train at all, I just go out and run." In the 1500 she trailed a much younger runner by about 4 strides for 3 laps and with about 100 metres to go on the last lap, she was able to overtake the younger runner and win by about 4 strides. It was so much fun to watch. She has a runner's body but she certainly didn't let age be a factor in whether to run or not. She just did it.

Also, there was a ninety-six-year-old golfer who I knew, who was competing at those games. His category was eighty and older and when he was ninety-five, he won gold for both the nine-hole and the eighteen-hole rounds. He had also attended the nationals and won gold for eighteen holes and silver for the 9-hole round. At ninety-five, he outplayed fellows who were as much as fifteen years younger than himself. It shows that if you are slim and fit, age doesn't matter. It's only a number.

And as we'll learn later, fitness and good health play a part in helping to slow the onset of Alzheimer's and Parkinson's. And who doesn't want to delay or avoid the onset of either one of those diseases?

In the next chapter, we'll also learn about the need to include squats in an exercise program. But for now, I want you to think about getting up off the toilet. It's something that everyone has to do every day. *Like it or not!* And as we age, we realize that it seems to be harder and harder to do. Landfill sites across the country are collecting many old toilets. Why? Because people are getting rid of old low-slung toilets and replacing them with modern taller ones. We've replaced the two in our house and it's remarkable how much easier it is to get back up from them compared to the lower ones. It's very obvious how much more difficult it is when we go somewhere else that has low toilets. But our strong leg muscles gained from squat exercises over the years, has made it much easier to get up and down from short or tall toilets.

Also, if you are a traveller and have been to Middle Eastern or some Asian or African countries, you know about the holes in the floor in many places where you might have to go to the washroom. There is no escaping it. No nice clean toilet to sit on. You don't want weak leg muscles when you squat there. I just can't imagine falling over in that environment because my leg muscles weren't strong enough to bring me out of the squat. Hence, we continue to work those muscles every time we do our exercises. And we may not go to those countries now at our age but many readers of this book, may still want to travel. Get fit I suggest and you'll never regret it. Even if you only stay at 5-star hotels. Being fit allows you to see more than you might if you are out of shape.

I have a strong desire to get my fitness instructor's certificate. Not only will it legitimize that I am serious about being fit as I grow older, I have decided that I want to be the one who conducts fitness classes at the next place where Bev and I might end up living. I want to be able to show folks how fitness can and will work for them. And I'll be able to make sure that their exercises are done correctly. I was sad to observe a middle-aged instructor, at an assisted living place, conducting exercises way too fast for the average age of the class she was teaching. Our former fitness instructor, Sharon says that when older folks exercise too fast they could end up with broken bones because some of them will undoubtedly have osteoporosis. I want to *know* my audience and treat them accordingly. Fitness, yes of course, but at a pace that is age appropriate. I plan to be that type of instructor in the future.

Dr. Blouw points out that a US cardiologist of the 1950s, Paul Dudley White of Harvard University, suggested that people should, "Eat less, walk more, and sleep more." 'And of course, this is still as true today as it was 70 years ago.'

And Dr. Blouw continues, "just walking is good enough, particularly when we age. Simply going at four miles per hour (a brisk walk) for half an hour, which would be two miles in distance, for five out of seven days per week, confers tremendous health benefits. It raises your good cholesterol, lowers your blood pressure, decreases anxiety and stress levels, burns off some blood sugar (a good thing, particularly if one has diabetes), and prevents the atrophy of muscles that occurs if a person is too sedentary. Weakened muscles can easily lead to falls and fractures. So, don't think of exercise as a weight-loss strategy, but as something to enhance the most valuable thing in your life…. your health!"

And Dr. Blouw goes on to say, "I focus on walking because it's easy to do, effective, and inexpensive. Many folks say they can't exercise because 'I don't have the time', but if it takes only thirty minutes per day, is there not a TV show or reading a tabloid or some other thing that could be sacrificed instead? Watch an hour of TV, instead of an hour and a half. Research has shown that folks who watch six hours of TV per day might *reduce* their lifespan by five years."

Wow, isn't that an impressive statistic? Just by sitting around watching TV for six hours every day can shorten your lifespan by five years. Doesn't just knowing that fact, motivate you to get up off the couch and get moving? As I said before, I didn't write this book to judge anyone's lifestyle, but I do want to point out to folks how my program worked for me over the years. And when a physician who has been in family practise for over 40 years, points out this information on being fit and living a healthier lifestyle, I have to sit up and take notice.

Once people retire, they have the time and more often than not, they have the money to do things that can help them live a healthier life style. But this certainly is not the time to let things slip away. There are fitness classes like Bev and I joined, there are gyms (post covid) where a person can go and get personal instruction on how to use the equipment there. Some folks hire a personal trainer who helps them develop a program that is right for them and helps them set reasonable and attainable goals. But really, if you're too shy to go out and be seen working out in front of others, just simply get up off the couch and start doing something. And as Dr. Blouw says, "walking does have wonderful health benefits." If you have access to a bike, that's a good way to get fresh air and work at getting fit. Over time you will build strength and endurance.

You've bought this book or it was given to you by someone who cares, so if you've gotten this far in reading it, then maybe you've come to understand that being fit has some merit for you in living a healthy lifestyle. It's really up to you. Think about it, take the necessary steps to get up off the couch and you'll be on your way to a healthier lifestyle.

The last word in this chapter goes to Dr. Blouw who says, "As the Nike commercial said; '*Just do it!*'"

"Exercise is a key component to both quality of life and longevity."

a slimmer you

TIPS FROM CHAPTER 8:

1. Being fit means you can do more.

2. Being fit means fewer health issues.

3. Walking is a good start.

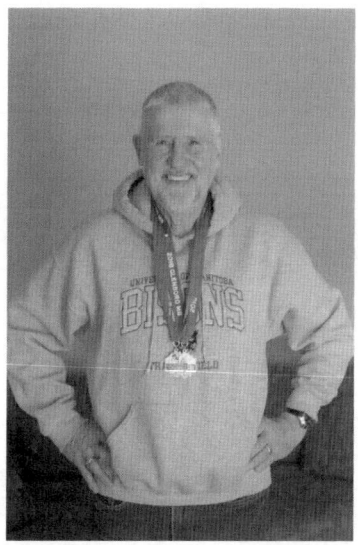

Gold medals at the 55+ Games - 2018 Glenboro, Man.

CHAPTER 9
Staying Fit

Many readers of this book will remember Ed Allen and several others may never have heard his name before. But before continuing this chapter on how to stay fit, I want to inform you a bit about Ed Allen. He was a TV host of his own program for a number of years when he decided that fitness should be important for everyone. So, over many years he filmed a series of TV episodes where he was seen practising and teaching calisthenics on a beach in different locations but mainly in California. However, he did shoot sixty-five episodes of thirty minutes each in southern Ontario. This was during the 1960's when many people considered that working out was something only sissies might do. In fact, good-ole farm boys like me, who watched Ed Allen, would sneer and say things like, "Why doesn't that guy get a real job?" Or, "doesn't that guy look dumb jumping around in that form fitting one-piece polyester jumpsuit?" There were several other comments as you can imagine.

To say that Ed Allen was ahead of his time would be an understatement. But he did have a loyal following and he didn't care what people said about him, he just went about his business. Besides he always had the last laugh. That's because in 1969, Ed Allen was pulling in $100,000 US a year. And that's the equivalent of well over $700,000 US annually in today's money. Not bad for a guy jumping around on a beach in a one-piece jumpsuit. And to put things into perspective, the average annual wage in Canada at the time was $5,893.76. And in today's dollars, that would be a salary of $42,630.51. So, it just shows how well Ed Allen understood fitness and what it could do for him and his television audience to say nothing about his bank account. Ed died in 2018 at the age of 92. It's not hard to visualize that his level of fitness over the years led to a long and healthy life for him.

From the last chapter we learned that there is no silver bullet to becoming fit. You have to work at it and it's easy to get started by getting up off the couch and simply going for a walk or a bike ride or to the pool for a swim. And as we've said, you don't need a gym membership to do any of those things. You just need to get moving.

However, on your way to getting fit, you want to exercise the muscles that may have been neglected for a while. In the last chapter we talked about how squats can help strengthen leg and lower body muscles to help you stand when getting up from a toilet seat. What are the muscles that we work when we practise our squats? First and foremost, we work the gluteus muscles which are a set of three that surround the buttocks. Then there are the quadriceps in the front of the thigh, the hamstrings which are in the back of the thigh, the calf muscles behind the lower leg, the adductor muscles in the groin area and hip flexor muscles that surround the hips. When we work those muscles by regularly doing squats, we strengthen them all and that keeps the lower part of our body strong.

We do push-ups to strengthen our chest muscles (pectorals), our shoulder muscles (deltoids), back of the arms (triceps) and the abdominals which are the muscles that surround the stomach area. Bicep curls are fairly obvious. When lifting weights or using a band or tubing for bicep curls, we strengthen our arm muscles and that helps us with our daily activities like carrying in groceries or lifting and carrying children. You also want strong arms for hoeing, raking, shovelling or any other chores where lifting or carrying is required.

Tricep muscles are found on the opposite side of the arm from the biceps and they control the movement of the elbows, the shoulders and the forearms. When you perform tricep kick-back exercises you strengthen the shoulder joints which are important to help you carry out any daily activity, but especially where arm movements are repetitively used in sports. Think of movements made with the arms in hockey, volleyball, tennis, basketball, or swimming. You want your triceps to be in top shape when participating in any one of those activities.

When you start to learn to do a plank exercise it seems to be the toughest of all exercises. That's because for most of us, holding our body weight straight up from our toes and onto our elbows isn't easy, especially if we haven't done it for a while or perhaps never. But with practise it becomes easier. Holding a plank position for a specified period of time, helps to improve body balance and posture, strengthens our core muscles, improves flexibility and over time will tighten the tummy muscles and help reduce belly fat. Also, over time you might notice that the constant backache that has been bothering you has started to lessen in intensity.

The abductor muscles around the hips, help us stand, and walk and easily rotate our legs. When these muscles get regular exercise, they help create a toned backside and can help to prevent pain in the hips and knees. They are related to the core muscles and help with balance and performance of athletic activities.

Adductors are a group of five muscles located in the thigh. They control the thigh bone's ability to move inward from side to side. They are commonly known as groin muscles. And if you've ever pulled a groin muscle, you know that it takes a long time to heal. I pulled one once just by kneeling down to get ready to throw a curling rock after Christmas. It hurt and I did not get physiotherapy right away, so the healing process took a long time. I now pay special attention when I do exercises for the adductors. I want to note here that we had been away from our exercise class for a month during Christmas break when I pulled the groin muscle. Now we exercise regularly in our basement, but I learned the hard way that a continuous exercise program is essential.

The latissimus dorsi muscles or *lats* are located on both sides of the neck just under the shoulder and they end up at the hips. They are the largest muscles in the upper body. They work when we open a car door, or pull on a strong door to open it. Lats really are involved in most of our daily activities. They're connected to the upper arms as well as the shoulder blades and down to the ribs and spine. They do a lot for us when we rotate our arm and pull things (like doors) towards us. Strong lats also contribute to how fast we can run, increased breathing potential and they provide strong support to our back.

Deltoid muscles or as they are commonly called *delts* surround the upper arm and shoulders. They support the movement of the arms and along with the biceps and triceps they help when we lift or pull objects.

The trapezius muscle is a large triangular shaped muscle that is found behind the neck which fans out in a triangular shape behind the shoulders and upper back. It works to tilt and turn our head and the neck, to shrug our shoulders and helps in twisting our arms.

All these muscles, plus many minor ones are important for our bodies to function properly. They all work to support strength and movement. I won't go into details about how to exercise each of these muscles, but if you want a fit body as you age, then you may want to learn how to do the proper exercises to strengthen those muscles. Our fitness instructor suggests 3 times a week for an hour each time. Some folks go to the gym every day but aging bodies need a break and three times a week is just fine to help maintain a fit body. If you follow an exercise regime that's right for your body and strength, you'll become more fit and that's important for you as you age. You'll feel better, you'll look better and you'll be able to lift and play with your grandchildren and maybe even your great grandchildren as you get older. Isn't that a wonderful goal to want to achieve?

But after having said all this about getting in shape, I want to caution you to check with your own family doctor to find out how much exercise you should be doing. Especially if you've been living a sedentary life and now want to get going. Your doctor has your health history and they can recommend what is right for you.

Bev and I started on our fitness journey back in 2005 when we went to visit my daughter Sarah and her now husband Steve, when they were living in Manchester, England. We had mentioned to them that if they stayed there for two years, we would go and visit them. But when our trip was being planned, we felt that we should try to get a little more fit. We were sure that Sarah would have us out hiking and climbing in the hills and moors of Scotland and we wanted to be able to endure the rigours of doing those activities.

Luckily, at about that time we got a flyer in the mail advertising a fitness course that we could sign up for at the University of Manitoba. The course was advertised as Resistance Training for Older Adults and we felt that it could fit the bill for us. It was the best thing we could have done. Our instructor turned out to be Sharon Couldwell, who was a fitness instructor for many years and the best instructor for people our age that a person could ever hope for. Sharon understands exactly what older people need to build strength, exercise the muscles and tone up the body. She is so gentle with everyone in the class. Sharon wants all participants to build up their body strength but only in a way that works for each individual. If you can't do as many reps as she is asking for, she encourages you to just do what you can. If you start with light weights, then over time she encourages you to step up to higher weights but only if your body agrees. If increased weights start to cause strain or pain, then Sharon gets you to back off. The class is designed to help people get stronger but only if you are comfortable doing so. Bev and I attended Sharon's class in the spring of 2005 and enjoyed it so much that we signed up for her classes and attended regularly for the next fifteen years. We were surrounded by like-minded folks who were at least our age or older. They all were attending because they realized the combined benefits of becoming fit and staying fit. Eventually, we realized what a social network we had acquired. A few in the class had been with Sharon for over the twenty-five years she'd been teaching there. And one lady named Sylvia was over 85 years old. I always told her that she was my role-model. And I meant it. Bev and I always thought that if Sylvia could get up and make it to class in -30 C weather, then there was no excuse for us not to do so.

Anyway, over the years I was able to increase my weights for bicep curls from eight pounds, up to ten, then twelve, and then fifteen and I was very happy when twenty-pound weights were added to our exercise room. I eagerly started using them and was planning to step up to twenty-two pounds when I began to experience sore elbows. When I confided that fact to Sharon, she told me to back off because my body was telling me that I was using weights that were too heavy for me. Now I use a combination of weights that total sixteen pounds and that seems to work. My elbows no longer experience pain. Going from eight to twenty pounds probably took more than a decade but it shows what a person can accomplish when they have a desire to get fit the proper way. I slowly got stronger and along with losing body fat I not only felt stronger but I finally liked the look I was seeing in the mirror.

Another thing that you should know is that Sharon never had us do a large number of reps at each exercise class. Twelve reps of one exercise, say lower body, followed by twelve reps of an upper body exercise and then back to the first one for twelve more reps. That's a total of twenty-four reps and that sequence was managed through all the exercises that we performed at each session. Each day began with ten minutes of warm-up, forty minutes of actual working hard followed by ten minutes of cool down. Perfect for us aging folks.

However, I want to point out something here. I had been going to exercise class for five years when I saw the picture of myself that sent me on my journey to lose weight. In other words, my body was already at a certain level of fitness. What I realized I needed to do was to lose weight and continue to be fit. And of course, it worked. You wouldn't be reading this book if the combination of fitness and weight loss hadn't helped me achieve my goals. Now, in my 70's I am more fit than I was in my 60's and I'm quite proud of the fact. It just feels right.

I asked Sharon if she would be willing to contribute to this book and she was more than willing. I was pleased and felt privileged to have her do so. Before including her comments, I want to point out that when the gym closed in March 2019 from Covid protocols, Sharon decided to retire. That was a sad moment as I was hoping she would instruct us until we could no longer attend. But she was such a good instructor over the years that I was able to learn enough to conduct our own exercise class in the basement of our house all through the Covid 19 pandemic. So, Bev and I are staying in shape by continuing to exercise for one hour three times a week, just like we did during Sharon's classes. And now let's hear from Sharon.

I started in the fitness industry in 1987. Initially I was looking for a way to improve my own level of fitness and to get back to the levels I had enjoyed when I was younger before having my children. I came from an athletic family and all during my school years I was always very active in sports. I missed the physical as well as the social aspects of team sports. I always enjoyed people and the social benefits of sports.

Firstly, I joined a fitness facility club and started as a participant. Fairly quickly I became disillusioned with the level of instruction and information provided. I knew there was more to fitness than what I was seeing in most classes. I wanted to know more. I wanted to know why a particular exercise was good for me and what it did for me. What muscle group was I working and why was that good for me. I wanted to learn more and started taking courses to become a certified fitness instructor. I took the courses and came away with a new knowledge and an eagerness to pass this on to other participants.

Once I got my credentials and started to teach, I found most participants were just like me and wanted more than just a physical workout; they also wanted to know why and what value they were gaining.

I have taught fitness professionally for over thirty years. Over these decades my greatest joy was to mentor participants into becoming more knowledgeable and making fitness a lifelong goal. Many participants even went on to become fitness instructors themselves. People start with short term goals, getting a little more fit for travel or keeping up with friends and family or perhaps recovering from a health problem. Fortunately, many of these short termers quickly saw the benefits of a fitness lifestyle and became permanent long-term members of my classes. I am constantly being reminded of how these transformations have improved quality of life, both mentally and physically, for the participants. I've watched them gain higher levels of energy and improved mental capacity.

Another big part of fitness training is the social aspects of joining a group. Members develop new long-term friendships. They meet new people and enjoy the company of like-minded people.

Teaching fitness has been truly a joy and if you enjoy what you are doing you will never work a day in your life.

It was a pleasure to add Sharon's comments to this book. Everything she states here is what all of us who attended her classes have felt for a long time. And we've all appreciated the efforts that she has put in over the years to help get us fit and to look better and feel better about ourselves.

The journey for me has taken a number of years but there is a level of joy that I've experienced as I realize that what I've steadily worked at has actually paid off. Looking better and feeling better is just a bonus to losing weight and staying fit.

But many people might say, "So what's the big deal?" And my answer to that question is simple. There are so many things I can do at my age that I never thought would ever be possible. Like running good times in the 55+ Games sprint races, like getting through harvest without experiencing aches or pains, like playing soccer with grandkids without getting out of breath. All these things and more have led to what I feel is a very good lifestyle and I want it to continue as I grow older.

But I want you to remember that it's a long-term undertaking of losing weight slowly, of eating all of your favourite foods (just less of them at each meal), of managing your food intake, of relying on your scale daily, and of maintaining a level of fitness that is definitely right for you. It seems like a lot, but the rewards are tremendous. Your family will appreciate what you've done and you'll be a lot healthier to play with grandchildren and perhaps great-grandchildren. Pictures of you doing that are priceless. How do you put a dollar figure on those type of results? I don't believe you can.

If you follow an exercise regime that is right for your body and strength, you'll become more fit and that's important for you as you age.

TIPS FOR CHAPTER 9:

1. Staying fit takes a degree of effort.

2. Strong muscles mean a fit body.

3. Benefits of being fit are numerous.

a slimmer you

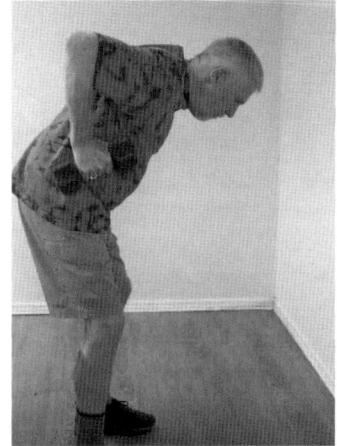
Dumbbell row

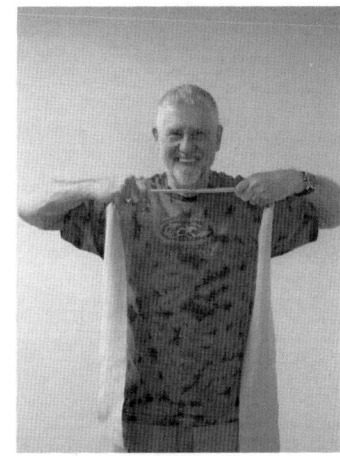
Posture muscle exercise

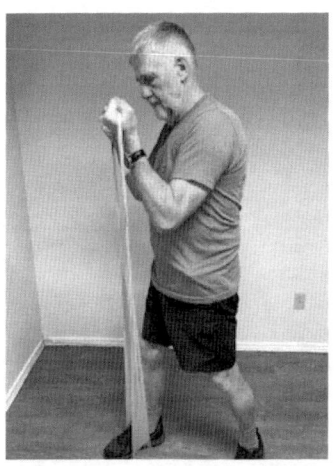
Bicep curls with band

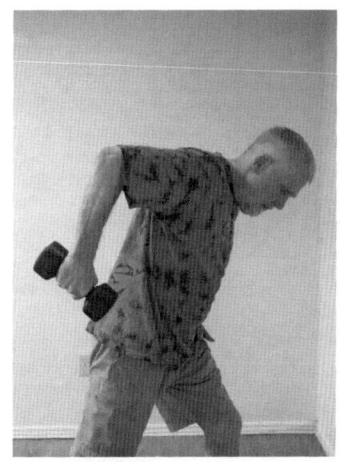
Tricep exercise

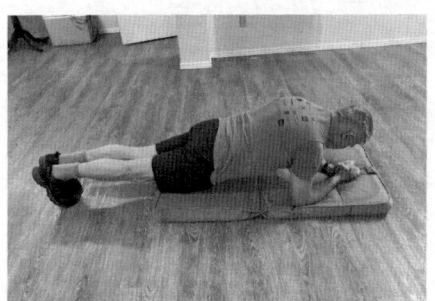
Holding a plank position

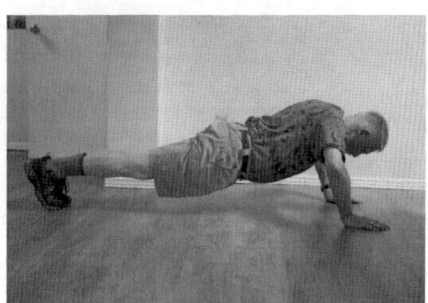
Push-ups exercise

CHAPTER 10
The Value of Core Strength

In the chapters on getting and staying fit, you learned about why I decided to get fit and how I accomplished my goals. We mentioned core strength in the chapter but didn't really describe what it is and why it is important.

So, what is core, where are the core muscles, and why is it important to have strong core muscles? Core muscles are those muscles that support the body in several ways. They enable us to have strength and to twist, to lift, to turn our bodies in ways that do not injure us. Although they're throughout the body, along the spine for instance, core muscles mainly exist around our lower body and especially the stomach and back areas of the body.

Think about top level athletes. They're able to achieve what they do because they have very strong core muscles. If they didn't, it would be impossible for them to compete in their sport at the highest level of competition and endurance. In reality, think of any athlete and what they are able to accomplish. Be it hockey, figure skating, ballet, martial arts, football, running, curling, rock climbing and anything else you can think of, what is the one constant with all of them? It's that all these athletes have worked hard to strengthen and maintain their core muscles.

We've all heard of abdominal muscles (abs), we've heard of oblique muscles, we've heard of many different muscles in our body with names we might not recognize. But they all exist and they allow us to perform our daily movements. In fact, there are twenty-nine main muscles that make up our core. Some are more evident and you can feel them when you pull up your tummy and others are hidden deep and surround our inner skeleton. But every single one of them is there to help us complete our daily tasks. Without them, our skeleton would just slump in a corner, going nowhere.

One of the most important muscles is the quadratus lumborum muscle. You don't have to remember this name, but it's important for you to know that it exists and is commonly referred to as the QL muscle. This muscle is found on both sides of our body at the back. It is our deepest abdominal muscle and we often hear it referred to as the back muscle. And that is the one that is most affected when friends or family say they've got a bad back. When people experience lower back pain, it's often due to muscle fatigue and shows up when you're sitting too long, such as at a computer or riding in your car.

Core muscles help us to do simple things like bending over but really, think about everything else you do in a day. It starts when you get out of bed in the morning and continues throughout the day. Walking, lifting, running, opening doors, walking up and down stairs, carrying groceries, lifting or playing with children, driving your car and even typing on your computer involves your core muscles. And I believe that it's important to keep your core muscles tuned up (toned up) just like it's important to keep your car tuned up. In the case of your car, when it wears out you can get a new one and keep going wherever you desire to go. Unfortunately, it's not possible to go out and buy a new body, but if you keep the one you have tuned up, then it will last you a lot longer before it starts to run down. And that is the essence of *A Slimmer You*. When you've lost unnecessary weight and you've learned to tune up your core muscles, you will experience a stronger, healthier body that is able to accomplish daily tasks with ease.

Fitness experts claim that underworked core muscles start to deteriorate after a few weeks of reduced activity. You may not notice it happen but it could show up eventually with a bad back, strained ligaments or worse. Staying fit can ready you for a healthy future and is the cheapest form of insurance to get you there.

And once you get into a routine, it only takes three times a week for us older folks to maintain a healthy body. Others may not notice that you are fit but they will notice that you are hardly ever ill and that you don't need to visit your doctor or a chiropractor very often. And eventually, they will also notice that you are walking tall and seem to have good posture compared to themselves. This all is the result of having a strong core.

When I think about core muscles, I clearly remember one time at the curling rink when I was putting on my curling shoes and I heard a conversation that went like this: "Did you hear about Joe?" Bill asked his friend. "No, but I did notice that he wasn't here last week," was the reply. "Well, it's very sad but when Joe bent down to tie his shoelaces, his back went out. Now he can barely walk."

Through the years, I'd heard the phrase "so and so's back went out." Over time, I was curious to find out what the cause was. And because I never knew for sure what happened to Joe's back, when I went to my next exercise class, I asked Sharon if she could tell me what had happened to Joe's back. Without hesitation, she said, "Joe's core muscles weren't strong enough to support the simple movement of him bending over to tie his shoelaces." She went on to explain that if Joe had been doing regular exercises to strengthen his core muscles (like we do in our classes), then he might not have gone down with a bad back.

Remember the quadratus lumborum (QL) muscle that we just talked about? That's the one that causes much of the lower back pain that people experience. Chiropractors and masseuses must love the QL muscles. Think about it! Where do many folks go when they experience lower back pain? They go to see their chiropractor or their massage therapist to get relief. It hurts so much that they must do something. Or they visit their doctor to get a prescription for drugs to help them deal with the pain. And they do get relief. However, without regular exercise to strengthen the core muscles, they'll need to return to the chiropractor or massage therapist to help correct another bad back. Or they'll have to rely on over the counter or prescription drugs. That's because every day we are all required to perform a number of functions where we need to use our core muscles. Those muscles have to be able to handle it. Like so many other things, quality of life increases when we can do all the normal, everyday things without worrying about our back "going out."

When we have strong core strength, we can easily do so many of the things we've always done. Isn't it great to be able to carry in the groceries with ease, to push open heavy doors without straining too much, maybe to build a deck in the back yard or at the cottage at the lake? All these are possible into our old age if our core is strong enough to handle these tasks.

I have found that because of improved core strength I can lift heavy items and do necessary chores a lot easier than I used to be able to do. Even as recently as ten years ago, I used to find that moving three heavy batteries in and out of my boat every year was a tough task. I grunted and groaned and questioned whether I should be selling the boat or not. Now with a stronger core, I can complete that task much easier. And I've worked at either operating a combine or driving a grain truck at harvest every year since 2002. You've read how I love being out in the fields at harvest. And I'm sure you know how important it is to be fit when working on a farm at harvest. Shedding extra pounds and strengthening my core muscles has enabled me to get through each season's harvest with minimal physical discomfort.

And during any given harvest season, as I've said before, I will be in and out of either a truck, a combine or a tractor over 500 times. That's a lot of stepping up and down. Imagine what shape my body might be in if I didn't have strong core muscles or I still weighed 185 pounds. I do this every year because, when I grew up on the farm, harvest was the most fun of any season for me. It's always a challenge to get the crop in the bins before the weather changes and I forever enjoy the buzz of harvest time. Now it's even more fun when I can be around and work with big equipment that I don't have to own, maintain or pay for. And I'm so grateful to have strong core muscles that help me be out there and complete all my required harvest tasks.

A healthy core means I can lift my grandkids, play games with them, take them fishing and rough-house with them without fear that my back will "go out." In other words, it allows me to live the type of life I always imagined, as I thought about growing older.

By now maybe you'd like to know how to start to strengthen your own core muscles. Well, getting started is as easy as sitting in your chair and performing a simple exercise. All you have to do is tighten your tummy muscles and pull them up towards your rib cage. Hold them in that position for a count of ten and then let them relax. Do that again for a count of ten and keep doing it until you've done it ten times. That will be enough for now but congratulations, you have just started to strengthen your core. You can do it sitting down or standing up or when you are going for a walk. Nobody will even know you are strengthening your core muscles, but you'll know. And when you're out walking, if you learn to consciously walk with your core muscles pulled in and tightened, you are on your way to a stronger core and you'll notice your walking posture changing. That's the good part of working on your core strength, there are little side benefits that you didn't even realize before.

Another way to strengthen core muscles is to get a five-foot long exercise band. They are cheap and flexible and you can get one at an exercise supply store or medical supplies store. They come in different colors denoting the strength that you might need for your ability. You can start with a more flexible band and move up to more powerful ones as your strength increases. An elderly person who wants to start to become more fit, needs the color that is best suited to their abilities. Someone younger and stronger might get the top-of-the-line stronger band. These bands can be used to work your posture muscles, your biceps, your triceps, and if you go to the floor, they can be used to work your hamstring muscles and also to perform low rows or high rows that will strengthen arm and back muscles. If these terms seem foreign to you, don't worry, just purchase an exercise book that will demonstrate how to use the band. Check online or, best of all, check with a fitness instructor. But remember not to overdo your exercises as you get started. Just take your time and stronger muscles will eventually develop.

You can also invest in weights that are suitable for your own abilities as they come in all sizes. But I caution you to consult your doctor or health practitioner if you have any medical issues, as they will be able to advise you on how much you should do to get started. I certainly do not want anyone to injure themselves when they first start out. That's the quickest way to abandon your goal of strengthening your core muscles. And I wouldn't want that to happen. I want you to experience a successful outcome.

So much starts and ends with good core strength and it pays dividends when your core is strong enough to support everything you do without having your back "go out." That includes carrying in groceries, lifting them up to empty the bag, lifting your children or grand-children, lifting your boat trailer hitch, shovelling snow, hammering or sawing for your new deck and any other movement that activates your core muscles. Core strength is essential to a long and happy future. With a strong core, you'll never regret all the rewards you'll get for having made the effort.

I believe that it's important to keep your core muscles tuned up (toned up) just like it's important to keep your car tuned up.

TIPS FROM CHAPTER 10:

1. A strong core helps our body in so many ways.

2. A strong core prevents our back from "going out".

3. Strengthening core muscles is relatively easy.

CHAPTER 11
How Bad is Belly Fat?

I've talked at length about how carrying extra weight (especially around the waist) can affect the present and future health of people. In this chapter I want to discuss what belly fat is and why it's a good idea to shed pounds for all the right reasons. We all carry a little extra fat and that's not a bad problem in and of itself. It's certainly OK to have a little extra weight in reserve. Those additional pounds come in handy if we are hospitalized for a medical issue that puts us out of commission for a while. But extra weight is a problem if a person is overweight or obese.

Belly fat is described as excess fat in the lower body or stomach area, which is commonly called the belly. There are two main types of fat: subcutaneous fat and visceral fat, which accumulate in the lower abdomen. Subcutaneous fat lies just below the surface of the skin and visceral fat is located deeper in the body and surrounds all the organs. Subcutaneous fat looks bad when you see it in an overweight person but it's the deeper fat (visceral) that's of greatest concern. We know that being overweight can lead to health problems. However, it's important to know that the body needs a certain amount of visceral fat. It's there to surround and protect our inner organs.

But it really is extra visceral fat that can lead to higher blood pressure, to higher LDL (bad) cholesterol levels, to Type 2 diabetes, and to cardiovascular disease. And of course, when referring to cardiovascular disease, we need to be concerned about possible heart attacks or strokes.

Again, I want to state that I'm only presenting facts in this book and informing people about how my weight loss steps worked for me. I'm not a medical person, so I want to emphasize that your doctor can and should be the one to advise you on a weight loss program that is best for you. But I'm hoping that some of my methods help you attain your goals.

In looking up information for this chapter, I learned that men and women store fat in their bodies in different ways and I'll explain it as simply as I can.

For men: Men store fat in the abdominal area around their stomach. And mostly it's the aforementioned visceral fat that they store in their bodies. So, when you hear the expression that we've all heard before, "It's all bought and paid for," a proud fellow is referring to the extra fat around his waist that is commonly referred to as his beer belly. And more often than not that beer belly is there because of the number of beers that have been consumed in a person's lifetime. And often, it's a combination of consuming too much of the wrong type of food, bar food for instance, that goes along with the beer. Over a lifetime, the result of that type of lifestyle is simply too much fat. And for those who have never drunk alcoholic beverages but still have a *beer-belly*, it must have gotten there from consuming too many calories and not burning enough of them off.

For women: Research indicates that women store fat in their bodies differently than men. The reason is that women need a little more body fat to enable their bodies to carry and nurse babies. From what I've read, it appears that this difference starts when they develop as young women around puberty. Although not every woman goes on to have babies and raise a family, their body is hot-wired by nature to prepare for it. You've all heard the expressions for body shape as being pear-shaped or apple-shaped. Well, women tend to have more of a pear-shaped body, which is more evident as they get older. While that body shape is developing over time, subcutaneous fat is stored in the areas of the body such as the thighs, the hips, the buttocks, and the abdomen. But according to documents I've read, after menopause, the stored fat slowly changes from subcutaneous to visceral fat. Having a certain amount of this fat is actually healthy, but it's when a person carries too much visceral fat that problems arise.

Even while discussing the differences between men and women as far as stored fat is concerned, we all know there are many different body shapes and sizes. Our genetic make-up has already taken care of that. But what can be adjusted is the shape of that body if a person is carrying too much weight. So, if you really have a desire to slim down and to lose some of that belly fat, then I believe that now is the time to do something about it. And it's necessary to be realistic about your goals. We've talked before about how it has taken a lifetime to put on extra pounds that we don't need. So, a slow shedding of those pounds is the best policy, in my opinion.

You might recall that it took me three years to lose all the unneeded fat around *my own* belly.

No discussion about fat in our bodies is complete without discussing problems that too much trans-fat in our diets might cause. When extra trans-fat is consumed by eating a regular diet of fast foods like French-fries, hamburgers, fried chicken, fried noodles, battered fish, etc., then the body could be heading for trouble. It's too much trans-fat in the blood stream that leads to high cholesterol problems which can lead to clogging of the arteries. And that as we know, can lead to heart disease and stroke. Too much trans-fat can actually raise the levels of LDL cholesterol (or bad cholesterol) in the arteries and lower the levels of HDL (or good) cholesterol. And that might lead to high blood pressure, which means that folks are at greater risk of experiencing problems like the aforementioned heart attacks or strokes.

What are some solutions to preventing such an event in our bodies? Number one is to use moderation when eating fried foods (that we love and that taste so good). In other words, don't eat high trans-fat meals too often. Besides the heart and stroke problems, too much of a high trans-fat diet can lead to people developing Type 2 diabetes. We all know most of these facts, but a reminder doesn't hurt.

Do we know how much trans-fats are in the fake butter that goes on the popcorn that so many of us eat at the movie theatres? Among a number of ingredients is partially hydrogenated soybean oil (trans-fats) and buttery flavouring. This buttery flavouring is a chemical that's engineered to simulate real butter. When you enter a movie theatre, how can you resist those wonderful odours that associate movie watching with eating popcorn. And you know that the bigger the box, the cheaper the popcorn is so it's easy to eat lots of this "butter." Gotta have it!

It's important to learn to read labels, especially of processed foods you might buy for a quick and easy meal. It's easy to go over the daily limit of trans fats, especially when you notice that portion sizes listed are often much smaller than people might normally eat. For example, suppose the listed daily requirement of trans-fat of a particular food is for a portion size of 100 grams. That is quite common on labels. But what if a person normally eats four or five times that amount during the meal. It's easy to see how it's possible to exceed the daily level of trans-fats that are recommended for a healthy diet. And the same applies to sugar and salt as well.

As a counterbalance, plan to eat more healthy foods like fruits, vegetables, lean meats you cook yourself, whole grains, pulses like beans and lentils, fish, nuts, and lean poultry. Deli meats are good once in a while but they often contain too much trans-fat and or salt. Again, moderation is the key.

And of course, the best recommendation to counterbalance a diet that might include too much trans-fat or other ingredients, is to get up off the couch and get moving. It all helps.

In 2018 Public Health of Canada reported that 36.3 percent—or 9.9 million—Canadian adults were classified as being *overweight* and an additional 26.8 percent of Canadians (eighteen years and older) or about 7.3 million were classified as *obese*. Combined, that means that 63.1 percent of Canadians could (and many will) experience a negative health event as a result of being overweight.

According to the Public Health Agency of Canada, as of 2017, 30 percent of children aged five to seventeen were overweight or obese. That's almost a third of young people and that rate of childhood obesity has tripled since 1979.

So, how does this overweight situation even happen? With myself, the extra weight I was carrying just seemed to sneak up on me. Over several years during middle-age, the pounds slowly added on. One pound at a time. I didn't notice, I wasn't paying that much attention to my weight and I seemed to be healthy enough. I wasn't taking medication for any health problems and I felt that I was eating healthy enough food. But I realize now that I wasn't active enough and that I was consuming more calories a day than my body needed. Later on, even though I'd been attending exercise class for five years, it wasn't until I saw that picture taken by my friend Jim in 2009, that I realized I should do something about getting rid of that unneeded belly fat. Extra pounds that I realized I didn't need.

It dawned on me that eating too much, when I was no longer as active as I'd been when I was younger, was contributing to the extra fat I was carrying around. So, as you know I started to cut back on food intake, used the scale daily to monitor progress and along with exercise class, added all the other steps I mention in this book. However, what I recommend for *you* to get started is to check yourself in front of a full-length mirror. They are a cheap investment if you don't already have one. With your clothes off, turn sideways, take a look at your profile, and ask yourself. Am I happy with this look? If you aren't happy with what you see, then now is the time start to change that look.

I have friends who have told me that they are healthy and are doing fine. But I see myself in them. They have that "extra belly" that I know they don't need and they seem to be adding to it a bit every year. I know by looking at them that their *body mass index* readings have to put them into the overweight category. And, I would like to take a profile picture of them and suggest they read this book and start to follow the methods I've outlined. After all, it worked for me and I sure want to help them avoid future health problems. (We'll learn more about BMI readings in the next chapter.)

I may appear pushy, but I do want those friends around for a long time yet. You know as well as I do that you can't force people to change their habits. It's like trying to get someone to quit smoking or quit drinking too much alcohol. They have to seriously want to quit and no matter what their loved ones want them to do, it has to come from within. It's the same with folks who are carrying too much weight. They have to decide for themselves whether to lose their extra weight or not. No-one can force them to do so. I just hope this book might be a catalyst to get some readers motivated and to get them started on their own weight loss journey.

Why am I so concerned about my friends who carry extra belly fat? Well, we've discussed it before and we know that extra weight makes the heart work harder**.** We instinctively know that it's true. And we know that if the heart has to pump harder, then it's working overtime and, in most cases, has to beat faster. And, that often leads to higher blood pressure. I recently read, that women who are the most overweight, have a significantly higher risk of suffering a serious heart event than do women who weigh significantly less, or in other words, compared to women who are at a proper weight for their age, height and body shape. Heart issues may not necessarily happen to an overweight person, but carrying extra weight does increase the risk of a future cardiovascular event. (Heart attack or stroke). Results for men will be much the same because overweight is overweight. Carrying extra weight for anyone increases the risk.

I believe that it's important for overweight people to lose weight now to reduce the chance of dying too soon. It really is about length and quality of life. Too often I hear about people I know who have suffered a stroke and boy has that changed their lifestyle bigtime. It has been a gut-check journey for them as they've had to adjust to life in a wheelchair, reduced mobility, slower thought processing and a big reduction in things they used to be able to do. Things that were so easy for them just before their stroke. It really *is* about quality of life.

A statement from the newsroom at McGill University in 2014, stated that *"Obesity may shorten life expectancy up to eight years!"*

So, what can overweight people do to reduce the risk of having a heart event or a stroke? Almost every site on the internet about this topic recommends much the same thing. And the more I read on the topic, the more it looks like I've been on the right path with my weight loss program. It may even appear that I had read about all this before I started my journey back in 2010, but it's actually the other way around.

I accomplished what I did over the years and only started reading about all the benefits of what I've done when I decided to write this book. I've worked for over seventeen years with the resistance training program and with my weight loss strategies for the last twelve years. And now this year (2022), I've added to my knowledge about this topic from reading research papers and checking out a number of sites that offer the same advice as I've outlined in this book. I'm more than happy to know I've been on the correct path all along. And of course, all of this information is supported with solid advice from folks like retired family doctor Dr. Blouw and others.

Once again, these recommendations from the Public Health Agency of Canada punch home what I say throughout this book.

It's recommended that folks eat a healthy diet! *Check!*

It's wise to cut out sugary soda pop wherever possible! *Check!*

It's important to control portion sizes at the table! *Check!*

Some form of physical activity needs to be part of everyone's day! *Check!*

Try to quit smoking! *Check!*

I haven't been hitting too hard on the smoking bit, although most articles seem to state it over and over. It's a serious addiction and I know it's hard to give up the habit. But I think we all know that if a person is overweight and they smoke as well, that's a combined recipe for future health problems.

The bigger a person is, the greater the need for the heart to pump blood around to all the extra capillaries and areas of the body that need it. And with a greater strain on the heart, there is a greater chance of an ensuing increase in blood pressure. Too often high blood pressure leads to a heart attack or stroke. And that reality is greater for people who are overweight. It may be a tough concept to wrap one's head around, but it's true.

Also, to continue on the same repetitive theme, people need to eat well-balanced healthy meals, pay attention to the levels of salt, sugar and fat they consume, and see their health-care professionals for regular check-ups to monitor blood pressure, blood-sugar levels and cholesterol levels. In other words, people need to try hard to get healthy and stay healthy.

For your own sake and for your family, who want you around for a lot longer yet, plan to get moving. Get up off the couch, work in the garden, ride a bicycle, go for a walk and increase the speed and distance over time. Nothing is easy, but just go for it. And if you are like me, and attend senior games competitions, try to enter competitions that challenge you to the extent of your physical capabilities. It's a lot of fun and socially rewarding as well.

This advice isn't rocket-science, folks. It's all about becoming *A Slimmer You!* Not only a slimmer you, but a *healthier* you. Please do *something*. Your future depends on it.

I realized that eating too much, when I was no longer as active as I'd been when I was younger, was contributing to the extra fat I was carrying around.

TIPS FROM CHAPTER 11:

1. Belly fat accumulates in the lower abdomen.

2. Too much belly fat leads to health problems.

3. Pay attention to labels on processed food.

CHAPTER 12
We Aren't Created Equal

After reading everything I've written to date, I want you to know that I didn't just fall off a turnip truck. I'm not naïve enough to think that everyone is the same shape as me, has the same amount of weight to lose as I did or can be instantly successful just by cutting back on their intake of food. But I do believe that by employing some of these habits you can actually start to lose weight. However, in this chapter I want to address the differences that relate to you achieving your goals and what I did to achieve mine. A person can only manage what they can measure and we'll talk about those measurements

Have you ever heard of the acronym BMR? It stands for basal metabolic rate. And the definition of basal metabolic rate is simply the number of calories required to keep your body going while you are at rest. The lower your BMR then the fewer calories it takes to maintain your body at rest. The higher your BMR, the more calories are required to maintain your body at rest.

If you google basal metabolic weight, you will find a calculator that helps determine your own BMR. On April 12, 2021, when I punched my weight (158 pounds), height and age into the calculator, I found that my BMR was 1,411 on that day. But just to test the calculator, I used my same height and age but I made myself 250 pounds. All of a sudden, my BMR jumped to 1,984. That shows you the effect that different body weights have on BMR. But I know my BMR is higher than the 1,411 that the chart tells me. That's because I know that I am very warm blooded. I am the last one to put on a sweater when the weather turns cooler during the day. And I get very warm under the sheets, especially under flannelette sheets in the winter. So, you need to treat these BMR numbers as guidelines only. But if you're curious, punch in your own numbers. You may be surprised what you find. I have to mention that all these measurements are based on averages. In reality they give you a base-line for your own body and where you fit on the charts.

Another measurement of body health is BMI, or body mass index. It's defined as a person's weight in kilograms divided by their height in metres squared (kg/m2).

BMI measures the nutritional state of the body. In simple terms, it's a calculation of body fat. Once again you can find a calculator to determine your own BMI. When I entered my numbers to calculate my own BMI, my results came back at twenty-five. At 158 pounds, I am very close to being overweight but remember that I've held that weight for over nine years so I consider that to be a natural weight for me. Find the BMI calculator on the internet to find out where you fit on this chart. The information may help you with your decision to lose weight.

Below is the Stats Canada chart of different BMI rates and what it means to be at the respective levels. The information is from the Canadian Guidelines for Body Weight Classification in Adults.

BODY MASS INDEX – CLASSIFICATION TABLE

BMI (kg / m 2)	Classification	Risk of developing health problems
Less than 18.5	Underweight	Increased
18.5 to 24.9	Normal	Least
25.0 to 29.9	**Overweight**	Increased
30.0 to 34.9	**Obese**, Class I	**High**
35.0 to 39.9	**Obese**, Class II	**Very High**
40.0 or higher	**Obese**, Class III	**Extremely High**

I must point out again that BMI measurements and results as listed above are only guidelines and that they are helpful as a quick reading or marker as to where each individual stands. Proper assessments should only be taken by a health-care professional (doctor).

If your BMI is below *18.5,* you could be considered underweight. If that's the case, it may be showing certain health risks and you should seek medical advice.

If you decide to use the chart as a guideline for yourself then a BMI of between 18.5 and 24.9 is considered a healthy range for both men and women and that's the level where people are at the lowest risk of experiencing serious health conditions. A BMI between 25 and 29.9 is considered overweight. Over thirty is considered as being obese with three levels being identified.

According to the chart, I am considered overweight. Because of my fitness program, I don't believe I'm overweight at 158 pounds. And when I punch in a weight of 156 then my BMI reads twenty-four which is considered normal. Some days I actually weigh 156 pounds. It's important again to remember that these values are averages and vary from person to person.

With a BMI level *above 30*, a person is considered to be obese. And that means they are at increased risk for many diseases and health conditions, including heart disease, high blood pressure, Type 2 diabetes, breathing problems and more. They need to check with their doctor and consider how healthy eating and a proper fitness program can help to improve their overall health and quality of life.

Again, these readings do point out where an individual ranks when compared to the average. Although the BMI is a simple measurement, it does show whether a person is carrying too much weight or not. BMI can be useful to measure trends in population studies, but it should not be the only measurement to use to determine your ideal weight. Also, remember that one size doesn't fit everyone. We are all different because of our body shape and size, because of our age, and of course our level of fitness. But these measurements can help you determine your own level and perhaps help you set goals to become a healthier individual.

There is another measurement called BFI which is Body Fat Index. I only want to mention it here because I know some of you will find it on the internet. But I've checked it out and the calculator for it is so close in numbers to the BMI that it just might confuse you as it did me at the time. Stick with BMI for your own calculations and that should be sufficient.

I interviewed my nephew Tim Gompf when I decided to write this book. I hadn't seen him for a while when I ran into him in Brandon a few years ago. Right away I noticed that he'd lost weight and that he looked pretty darn good for having done so. I thought he'd shed a lot of pounds and I questioned him about his method. I was quite surprised to find that he hadn't lost a lot of weight, but he *had* lost weight strategically and got rid of extra pounds he no longer needed. When I quizzed him about what he'd done, these are some of his answers: "I cut out all pop. I never was much of a pop drinker but now I avoid it altogether. I quit drinking regular beer and all alcohol. I will have a non-alcoholic beer once in a while, but it has to be low in carbs. There are only a few brands that are low in carbs but I look for them every time."

Tim says he has reduced his intake of carbohydrates such as bread and potatoes and increased his consumption of berries, almonds, trail mix, and raw veggies. "I am very conscious of the number of carbs I eat every day," Tim admits. "I try not to go over fifty to sixty grams of carbs, but it once was common for me to be up around eighty or ninety grams every day. Once I lowered my carb intake, I started to lose weight." Tim pays attention to labels and makes sure he doesn't spend money on food and drinks that are loaded with carbs. He grinds his own salt at meals so he can easily control how much goes on his food. He knows how easy it is to go overboard with too much salt in his diet, especially in processed food. And like many of us, Tim agrees that as he gets older, his desire to eat big hefty meals has certainly decreased.

Tim's overall weight loss was just over 8 percent versus my own loss of 14.5 percent. But why did he look so good after just an 8 percent loss? It's because Tim has a big solid frame. He has broad shoulders and a deep chest. So, losing 8 percent of his body weight on his frame was enough to get him feeling good and looking good. He admits that his sons have slimmer body frames and if they were overweight, their weight-loss program would look a lot different. What I'm pointing out here is that every person has a different body shape and any weight-loss program has to be tailored to each individual. I know what has worked for me, and if you start with your own program, it might work for you as well. I may sound like a broken record but if you lose weight slowly, you'll be grateful for your accomplishments.

The weight-loss methods that I've outlined throughout this book can possibly be found on the internet now, but it's what I've been working at for twelve years. I've used information from many sources to pull all this into a straightforward format that is simple to read and easy to follow. It's a personalized account that has worked so successfully for me that I believe it can work for anyone. Once again, I urge you to start with a reasonable goal and mark that goal for some time in the future. Not thirty days, three months, or even six months. If you want to lose weight in the healthiest manner possible then I want to hammer home that a slow weight loss program is the key. Learn to manage your weight trends (either up or down) by using the scale every day. You can indeed eat all of your favourite foods (even desserts) if you just learn to manage the amount of food you eat every day. Smaller plate sizes can help.

Letting your dog lick your plate after eating may stop you from going back for seconds. Sure, I know that you could go and get another plate out of the cupboard and fill it up with seconds. But by letting the dog lick your plate it makes you think, "Do I really want to eat more food right now? Do I really *need* to eat more food right now?" With those thoughts in mind, then you know you really don't want or need to eat more. And you've reached a pinnacle in your weight loss program. You've really come to acknowledge that if you want to feel better, look better and defy the odds on a number of health problems, you have to initiate a program that will work best for you. I truly believe that this method is a very "common sense" way to lose weight and keep it off.

Now we've talked before about how taking a cruise might lead to increased weight gain because of all the delicious food that is always available on cruise ships. But this chapter is about how one size doesn't fit all of us. My body shape is different from yours, my nephew Tim's body size is different from mine, which is different from his son's shapes and will definitely be different from your own body size. That's why losing 14.5 percent of my starting point was good for me and left me looking and feeling better. And it allows me to do more things and to accomplish so much more than I could if I still weighed my original weight.

And that's why Tim looks and feels better by just losing 8 percent of his body weight. Your goals and weight loss will be different and I encourage you to get started and to stick with your plan. Consult your doctor about what you want to accomplish and how you want to do it. I'd be willing to bet that they will give you a green light to begin. But be sure to share with your doctor the steps I've outlined, to inform them of how you plan to reach your goals. In a few years I'm sure you will be congratulated by folks closest to you as they observe what you've accomplished. Stick with it, I know you can do it!

We all know that everything that I've outlined here is not magic and there are no overnight successes. A number of years ago, I heard an interview with Michael Bublé on the radio. He's a popular Canadian singer, songwriter, and record producer. He's been very successful and is recognized nationally and internationally. The host was quizzing him about how he had become an overnight success. At that time most people hadn't heard much about Michael

Bublé and yet he was rising quickly on the charts. His very quick answer was, "Look, I'm thirty-one years old, I've been playing in bars and lounges around the country since I was sixteen. If you call fifteen years of slogging in the trenches an overnight success, I guess you'd say that's it!"

It's the same with any successful athlete like Wayne Gretzky or Connor McDavid. Their natural talent is undeniable. They rose to the top because of that talent and because they were and are doing exactly what they wanted to be doing. In other words, they worked at it. They put in their 10,000 hours of work to reach their goals. And you know that weight loss just doesn't happen. You won't be an overnight success but if you stick with your plan, you will get the results you are looking for. There are several roads you can head down and you want to make sure you head down the one that will have you reach your natural body weight. You won't regret it.

And as Robert Frost so eloquently ended his poem "The Road Not Taken":

> Two roads diverged in a wood, and I—
>
> I took the one less traveled by,
>
> And that has made all the difference.

So, I encourage you to please choose the correct road.

If you want to lose weight in the healthiest manner possible then a slow weight loss program is the key.

TIPS FROM CHAPTER 12:

1. Check your own BMI level.

2. Weight loss is not a "one-size-fits-all" scenario.

3. Losing weight slowly is the only way to go.

CHAPTER 13
The Value of Proper Nutrition

We've talked a lot about losing weight and becoming fit. Make no mistake, these topics are the most important chapters in this book. But it's imperative to pay attention to our dietary choices when we discuss eating less food at each meal. If a person eats the wrong foods at the table, then eating less of them might not show on the scale. When I mention the wrong foods, I refer to many processed foods that often contain too much salt, sugar or fat. I believe it's important to know the value of healthy food versus unhealthy food. Sadly, many people just don't know the difference or care enough to know the difference. So, we'll address those differences and confirm how making good choices can help you achieve your weight loss goals. But first I have to enter a quote that most of us have heard many times, "Eat local, eat fresh, and never eat anything that your great grandmother wouldn't recognize." Hopefully, that statement will become clearer when we address the value of eating proper foods.

There is no reason for most people our age not to eat healthy foods. Why? Because a majority of us don't need to scrimp and save anymore. We have the money to shop at our favourite grocery store, at the local farmers' market or to buy direct from a nearby farmer and to pay a good price for quality produce. But many people choose to buy food that has been picked early and shipped halfway across the continent to land on our store shelves a few days later. Often it is cheaper than local produce so it becomes the product of choice in our shopping carts. Or many consumers go for the convenience of packaged food that just needs to be heated up—food that is often full of too much salt, sugar, or fat, or combinations of all three.

Now don't get me wrong, we all know that living in Canada, often it's necessary to buy fresh produce that *has* been shipped a long distance just because for many months of the year our land is non-productive. So, as shoppers we need to look at which fruits and vegetables are the freshest. And aren't we fortunate to be able to do so? Our parents had to can vegetables and fruits to last through the winters because fresh food just wasn't available at that time of year. And those canning processes took days in hot kitchens and hours of labour-intensive work. But our mothers and grandmothers took on that work to provide their families with the best food, in winter, as was possible. Aren't we fortunate now to be able to run to our local grocery store around the corner or in our closest town and pick up what we need and prepare a healthy meal shortly after we arrive home?

Before continuing, I believe it's important to point out that eating regularly is a necessary step in living a healthy lifestyle. And what I mean is that when a person's body gets used to eating three square meals at a regular time every day, then it's just like eating the right amount of food and staying fit. It becomes the norm for your system and contributes to an overall healthier body. And now I will share this true story about myself.

Many years ago, when we were much younger and going to bars on a Friday night, my then wife and I met a young traveller from Germany. Over the course of the evening, we invited him to stay with us. In the morning we offered him breakfast and he accepted. We took the time to sit down and enjoy the meal with him. When we revealed to him that we hardly ever ate breakfast, without hesitation, he said, "You're just too lazy to be bothered to make breakfast and sit down and eat it. You should be eating breakfast." I was taken aback. I thought to myself, *How could a house guest suggest such a thing to us?* But at the time, I just accepted what he'd said. We didn't change our eating habit then, but I know now that he was right. When you eat regularly and don't skip meals, it's easier to stick to a meal plan that is healthy for your body.

And besides, many of you may have heard of the word *hangry*. That's the term that's used when a person gets irritable and easily flies off the handle in anger for no other reason than that they are hungry. In other words, their body is telling them that it's past the normal time to eat. My wife Bev gets that way when a meal is late so it's important that we eat at regular times in our home. And that's good for my overall health. Bev says her grandfather would get the same way and her grandmother, who recognized the symptoms, would simply say, "It's time to feed the beast." So just remember when you are around a person who gets unnecessarily cranky if a meal is late, make sure to avoid an unnecessary confrontation and simply put on the feedbag.

The supplement business is big business and I know most proponents of supplements won't like to hear that for the most part they are unnecessary. For the longest time Bev and I have felt that if you eat proper and healthy foods then you'll get all the nutrients, vitamins and minerals that your body needs. That's right. This knowledge is not hidden under a box somewhere, and we know that dietitians everywhere have been promoting healthy eating for a very long time.

But many people feel they have to take supplements because they *think* (or have been convinced) that they aren't getting enough nutrients from their food. When I checked the value of the supplement business, nationally, in the US, and globally, I found varying numbers. But as close as I can determine, the business generates around $3 billion US a year in Canada, $35 billion in the United States and $140 billion globally in gross revenue every year. Continued growth is projected to lift the global value to around $280 billion US by 2028. That's in a few short years, folks.

Most people don't need to take supplements but of course there are exceptions. As I said, my wife Bev and I believe that we get what we need by eating a healthy balanced diet. And that includes the required levels of fats, vitamins, proteins, carbohydrates, minerals, fibre, and a healthy amount of water daily. And we also believe that the diet we eat provides us with all those essential nutrients at the required levels to keep us healthy. And those required benefits are achieved by eating a variety of foods.

When you're willing to make the effort to plan, prepare, and cook a variety of healthy foods, then your body will also benefit from the nutrients that a balanced diet provides. As we've said previously, eating nutritious meals at regular times is a good habit to cultivate. It's not good for anyone's system to skip meals. Perhaps we all did that during our working careers. But it's not considered a good habit to get into because our bodies need to be refuelled. And we all know what happens when we skip a meal. Say it's lunch that we've skipped. By the time late afternoon rolls around, we are super hungry. We either snack heavily before our evening meal and then fill our plates again at dinnertime (or suppertime if you'd rather call it that) or we wait it out and devour everything in sight. That's not a healthy way to enjoy food and it's certainly not good for our systems. When we eat at regular times and eat well-planned nutritious meals, our bodies appreciate that and treat us accordingly. It stands to reason that our body will function well and regularly when it's fed the food it requires at a regular time of day.

Also, I believe it's imperative that people learn to read labels especially on prepared food that you buy off the shelf. It's necessary to watch for high levels of salt, and fat and calories. And you must pay attention to the percentage daily value (DV) listed on food labels and also to the serving size. If the ingredient list says that these daily values are based on 100 grams of a serving and you eat 300 grams or more then you have to do the math. As a quick example, if a serving of ham is listed as providing you with 25 percent of your Daily Value (DV) of sodium and you eat four times that amount then you are at 100 percent of your daily requirement of salt. But that is only one meal and a portion of what's on that plate. You may have added salt to your veggies to make them taste a bit better. In this case, when you add the sodium that's present from your other meals for the day, you see how easy it is to exceed your daily salt requirement. And the same is true for the fats (especially trans-fats) and in particular with the sugars, which are listed in grams and displayed in calories. The labels don't normally list the daily values for the sugars, but I believe they should. They often do list the quantities of sugar in the food or drinks but for some reason they aren't required to tell you what percent of daily value for your body that is. However, some dieticians and nutritionists want that changed.

And when it comes to aforementioned ham (for those of us who eat it), it's important to read the sodium levels that each brand lists on their ingredient list as a daily value. I've checked and a small serving of ham can vary from a low of around 19 percent to a high of 45 percent of your daily requirement. So, it's easy to go over your daily requirement by eating two or three slices, especially of the high-sodium level brands. Which we often do simply because it tastes so good. Again, I suggest that you learn to check labels when choosing food for your shopping cart.

In searching for information about eating healthy, I turned to the most recent Canada Food Guide. There is a ton of information in the guide so in the interest of space, I am going to touch on some highlights and recommend that you check out the guide for further information.

On the first page, the guide states that: *Nutritious foods are the foundation for healthy eating. And vegetables, fruit, whole grains, and protein foods should be consumed regularly. Among recommended protein foods, are legumes, nuts, seeds, tofu, fortified soy beverage, fish, shellfish, eggs, poultry, lean red meat, lower fat milk, lower fat yogurts, lower fat kefir, and cheeses that are lower in fat and sodium. And foods that contain mostly unsaturated fat should replace foods that contain mostly saturated fat. It's important that people who want to eat healthier, study and learn what foods contain unsaturated fats and which ones contain mostly saturated fat.* And in this last version, the Food Guide recommends that water should be the beverage of choice.

Foods that Bev and I enjoy that are highly recommended are potatoes, blueberries (that we pick in the wild every year), and eggs, which we eat in one form or another as many as five times a week. (But only one at each sitting!) Potatoes are full of many required vitamins and minerals. Blueberries are loaded with antioxidants that help the body stay healthy. As well as being high in protein, eggs—and in particular the yolk—are high in vitamins, minerals, and nutrients.

Fish such as salmon is also a good source of protein as well as providing vitamins and minerals. Shellfish like scallops, mussels, oysters and clams are high in vitamin B12 and zinc. Kale is reported to contain high levels of minerals and vitamins and other healthy compounds but it's not a product that hits my plate very often. It's an acquired taste that I haven't quite gotten around to acquiring yet. But it's a healthy food for you to consider for your weight loss diet.

When it comes to drinks, the Canada Food Guide is quite adamant about pointing out the harm that constant consumption of sugary drinks can do to the body. I know a number of people, including our son-in-law Steve, who used to consume a lot of pop. But when these folks decided to cut it from their diet, they were able to shed pounds over time. And they never went back. Here's what the Canada Food Guide says: *Sugary drinks are beverages that can contribute to excess free sugars when consumed regularly. These include soft drinks, fruit-flavoured drinks, 100 percent fruit juice, flavoured waters with added sugars, sport and energy drinks, and other sweetened hot or cold beverages, such as iced tea, cold coffee beverages, sweetened milks, and sweetened plant-based beverages. While 100 percent fruit juice, sweetened milks or fortified soy beverage provide nutrients to the diet, these products can increase the intake of free sugars. Water, unsweetened milk or fortified soy beverage, and fruit should be offered instead. Sugary drinks should not be consumed regularly. In 2015, sugary drinks were the main sources of total sugars in the diets of many Canadians, with children and adolescents (nine to eighteen years of age) having the highest average daily intake.*

Sadly, many children go to school every day with a can of soda pop in their lunch bag. That to me is a sad situation that leads to an unhealthy body over time and a disaster in their mouth. I'm quite certain that dentists don't pack a can of pop in their own child's lunch bag.

Again, from the Food Guide: *Promoting the consumption of water instead of sugary drinks, and reducing the intake of confections (like candy) to a minimum, are important ways to help Canadians decrease free sugars intake and reduce the risk of obesity, Type 2 diabetes, and dental decay. Nutritious foods to consume regularly can be fresh, frozen, canned, or dried. Nutritious foods to encourage people to eat should have little to no added sodium and saturated fat, and little to no free sugars.*

Michael Pollan is an author who has written extensively about food. His books include *The Omnivore's Dilemma, In Defense of Food, Cooked, Food Rules, The Botany of Desire* and several more. From the book *In Defense of Food*, we have some wonderful quotes:

Don't eat anything your great-grandmother wouldn't recognize as food.

Don't eat anything with more than five ingredients, or ingredients you can't pronounce.

Stay out of the middle of the supermarket; shop on the perimeter of the store. Real food tends to be on the outer edge of the store near the loading docks, where it can be replaced with fresh foods when it goes bad.

Don't eat anything that won't eventually rot. "There are exceptions—honey—but as a rule, things like Twinkies that never go bad aren't food," Pollan says.

It is not just what you eat but how you eat. "Always leave the table a little hungry," Pollan says. "Many cultures have rules that you stop eating before you are full. In Japan, they say eat until you are four-fifths full. Islamic culture has a similar rule, and in German culture they say, 'Tie off the sack before it's full.'"

Families traditionally ate together, around a table and not around a TV, at regular meal times. It's a good tradition. Enjoy meals with the people you love.

From the fifth quote above, about leaving the table a little hungry. Isn't that how this book came to be, with an inspirational comment by Jackrabbit Johannsen about pushing away from the table? Anyway, this chapter is about eating healthy and if you start to control the amount of food you eat, keep track of your weight, and begin to get fit, you will notice your weight dropping in a most natural way. Know the value of nutritious foods and learn to check labels at the grocery store and to look for the varying levels of sugars, salt and saturated fats in foods, especially in processed foods. Learn to be food aware.

I'm not saying that that you shouldn't have the occasional hamburger from a fast-food establishment, or an order of Chinese food or a pizza prepared outside your home. Occasionally for a treat, we do that ourselves. And it feels good and tastes good. But if you make that a daily undertaking, then you'll be heading for weight gain and your goal of losing weight and keeping it off will only be a pipe-dream! So, it's important to recognize and learn how proper nutrition can help you in the long run. Life is a long-term proposition and isn't it important for you to want to continue your life in the healthiest way possible? You'll be happier, you'll look good, and you'll feel good as well. The choice is yours!

Many consumers go for the convenience of packaged food that is often full of too much salt, sugar, or fat or combinations of all three.

TIPS FROM CHAPTER 13:

1. Stick with healthy foods.

2. Learn to check labels closely.

3. Become more food aware.

CHAPTER 14

Three Renegades of Processed Food

To write this chapter I re-read a very interesting book by author Michael Moss. It's called *Salt Sugar Fat* with a sub-title of *How the Food Giants Hooked Us*. It's a very interesting read if you want to learn more about how manufacturers of processed foods get people to buy and enjoy the food in a package that's ready prepared and often contains too much of either sugar, fat or salt. Or combinations of two of these ingredients or even all three. The title of this chapter is not intended to make you believe that sugar, salt and fat in food are all bad and should be avoided at all cost. No, it's to help you understand how manipulation of these 3 ingredients in processed food that we buy, can lead us to consume very high levels of one or all of these ingredients. And of course, the end result often means that people go down a path of becoming overweight or even obese, which often leads to serious health events, as we've discussed in other chapters. All of which assist promoters of diet schemes. And the cycle continues.

Michael Moss was, for a number of years, an investigative reporter who has written for *The Wall Street Journal*, *New York Newsday*, *The Atlanta Journal-Constitution*, and, most recently, *The New York Times*. He won the Pulitzer Prize for exploratory reporting in 2010. Besides *Salt Sugar Fat*, he has written another book (2019) titled *Hooked*, where he delves into how food manufacturing companies cleverly work to get people *hooked* into continually buying their food. And how they've also purchased big *diet* companies (yes, that's correct) in order to profit from both helping people become overweight and also from helping them try to slim down. I hope to read this book soon, time-permitting.

What I learned from *Salt Sugar Fat* is how food companies work with focus groups to fine-tune the foods they prepare for sale. Chemists work hard in company labs to do the best they can to have food reach the *bliss* point for consumers. Moss explains that, "The bliss point is the precise amount of sweetness—no more, no less—that makes food and drink most enjoyable." Once that point is determined through studies in the lab with children (often between five and ten years old) or with adults, then food or drinks are created around that information. Focus groups are brought in to further refine the process. Little adjustments are made to add or subtract the amount of sugar or fat or salt that is being tested that day. The final amount of each ingredient in the processed food that goes to the market shelf, or cooler or freezer is determined by responses that people in the focus group have given. It's all a very sophisticated process.

When I learned all this, it got me thinking about what went on around food when I was growing up. Almost every farmer back then had a few milk cows and often farm survival revolved around selling cream to the local dairy which in our case was located in Brandon, Manitoba. Before my time, the cream cans were filled and taken to town where they were processed at the local creamery, later they were picked up and delivered to the dairy by train. In my time, a driver for the Brandon creamery stopped by twice a week to pick up the cream.

But separating the cream from the milk meant one thing. There was always fresh cream on hand. It went on cereal and was delicious on fresh fruit and on puddings. In other words, we consumed a lot of it. I was a skinny kid when I left home so what affect did the fat from all that cream have on me? None at all. I ate lots and often we had fatty roast beef or pork and we ate the fatty skin from chicken and turkey. Our dad George would always say, "This is the best part!" as he crunched down on a crispy skin of a freshly cooked chicken or turkey. We were so active on the farm back then that whatever we ate never showed up on our bodies. Our very good cook mum, Evelyn, never held us back from eating whatever she created in the kitchen and second helpings at any meal were the norm. Indeed, too much sugar, fat, or salt never entered the picture as long as the food tasted good. So, what's the difference in today's world?

Unfortunately, today, many of us don't burn off the extra calories that are present in much of the food we eat. The creators of processed foods don't really care about what or how much we consume as long as their sales continue. They know our bliss point and they do what they can to make sure that the food we buy "tastes good" and continues to move off the shelves. It's bottom-line driven and if people buy it and regularly eat it, who cares if they become overweight. Earlier, I touched on information from the book *Hooked,* where we learned that big food companies now own the big diet companies, as well. So, they've got you covered—both coming and going.

And those same companies don't worry about being under any obligation to create healthy foods that they sell. The bottom line is to make as much profit as they can while making the food taste good by twigging the different amounts of sugar, salt and fat in each portion. And with food valued at US$3 trillion of worldwide sales, you don't have to be an economist to see who controls what we put in our mouths. Or why. It's mind-boggling to say the least.

I know that different soda offerings as well as sports drinks and fruit drinks vary in the amount of sugar in each can, bottle or carton. I researched this topic by looking at labels and studying charts that list different amounts of sugar in each drink. It's hard to believe but even the smallest drink has as much as four teaspoons of sugar in it. Twelve ounces of different drinks vary from five teaspoons of sugar in sports drinks and vitamin-infused water up to *twelve* teaspoons of sugar. Apple juice might have ten teaspoons, sweetened bottled iced-tea eight teaspoons. Think of these numbers a different way. Would you really stir that amount of sugar into a cup of tea? Even adjusting for cup size, most people don't put more than two teaspoons of sugar into their tea or coffee. And ten teaspoons of sugar computes to 80 percent of a person's recommended daily intake. Drinking more than twelve ounces boosts the daily recommended amount of sugar even higher.

I read one statistic that suggests that if a daily drinker of a can of pop were to cut it out altogether, they could lose one pound of weight in three-and-a-half weeks. I know people who have cut out soda pop and lost weight while doing so. Our son-in-law Steve Melo stopped drinking coke after many years of consuming from 500 ml to one litre *every* day. Eventually, some of his liver enzymes rose to very high levels and his doctor recommended that he stop with the pop. He dramatically cut back his consumption and his liver enzyme level fell back to normal. About three or four years ago, he stopped with the coke altogether and doesn't miss it at all. He has felt much better since dropping that daily habit. Many other folks are also dropping sugary drinks. The alternative? Well, it's water of course.

And when Cristiano Ronaldo (at the Euro 2020 back in June 2021) pushed aside two bottles of Coke that were strategically placed on the podium beside him, and said "drink water," the share prices of Coca-Cola dropped by 1.6 percent, or the equivalent of US$4 billion. That's a fairly big hit money-wise but don't worry about the company going broke folks, their share prices returned to normal by the end of the same day.

Back when I was raising my four girls, we tried to limit the amount of sugar they were eating so we didn't put extra sugar on the cereals we provided for them. One time (later in life), my oldest daughter Laura admitted to me that she liked going to stay overnight with Grandpa and Grandma Gompf because Grandpa always put sugar on her cereal in the morning and it tasted better. I was not surprised about that because that was the norm when I was growing up. It's also a prerogative of grandparents to spoil their grandkids with sweets and send them home.

When it comes to the fat part of salt, sugar, fat, it's astounding what has been done with cheese. From the book, I learned that consumption in America of cheese or cheese-like products has tripled since the early 1970s. And Michael Moss writes, "Cheese has become the single largest source of saturated fat in the American diet. Day in and day out, Americans on average are exceeding the recommended maximum by more than 50 percent." Along with high consumption of sugary drinks it's easy to see how the daily calorie intake of folks is at a very high level of 3,770. And lest we think ourselves smug, Canadians consume an average of a little over 3,400 calories a day. What happens to those extra calories when an average person needs only 2,000 calories to maintain a healthy lifestyle? Those extra calories get stored as fat in the body and lead to health problems we continue to mention in this book.

But how did we get to this stage? It's easy to explain. Back in the 1970's there was a big push to reduce fat in people's diets so it was decided that the fat in milk had to be reduced. It started by reducing whole milk (3.25 percent butter fat) down to 2 percent, then offering 1 percent, followed by skim milk. (Which in my opinion is nothing more that coloured water.) The switch-over with milk happened but it created a dilemma. What to do with the extra fat that was removed? That's when food manufacturers got creative. They offered a ton of different products that were cheese-enhanced and it was at that time that the pizza industry in America really took off. Who doesn't like a pizza loaded with all kinds of goodies and topped off with gobs of stringy, melted mozzarella cheese? And that's basically what became of the fat that was stripped out of milk.

But how are high levels of fat incorporated into food without us knowing it's there? It's because food chemists go to work to make sure once again that food is alluring to the taste buds. These researchers studied the sensory power of food and discovered that fat is about feel and texture in the mouth. So, when companies are told that they have to reduce the amount of sugar or salt in foods, they might do that but then increase the amount of fat in the food to keep its taste from failing. Consumers of food can taste if food is too sweet or has too much salt but there can be higher levels of fat in food and consumers can't and don't necessarily pick up on it. Unless they are strict label watchers like my nephew Tim.

Food labeling started to be mandatory around 1973, when consumers began demanding more information about the food they were buying, especially on labels of processed and packaged foods. So, the FDA in the US set about to establish rules and regulations about many of the ingredients you see on labels today. They are based on an average or usual portion size. If a person eats more than the recommended amount on the label, then they must adjust in their mind what they are actually eating. For example, if 100 grams of ham lists 35 percent of your daily salt requirement and you eat three hundred grams then you know you've exceeded your recommended limit of salt for the day. Reading labels can be painstaking and time consuming but we have to know what we are putting in our bodies and the bodies of our kids. However, what percent of the population actually reads labels? Many folks don't want to know that they are exceeding the recommended levels of sugar, salt and fats in the foods they eat. As long as the food tastes good to them and fills them up, what more do they need? This isn't a condemnation, it's just a reality for many consumers. And it's the taste-good level or "bliss" point that food manufacturers want you to have and to enjoy. Because for them it's mainly about the bottom line and you know the current slogan for anyone making and selling any product today, "It's because the shareholders are demanding it!"

I want to share one more story about cream. A friend of mine, Glen, told me about visiting an aunt when he was young. She always put on a wonderful spread at mealtime, which everyone enjoyed immensely. After some length of time, he asked his mum why her sister's food always tasted just a little better than at home. He was told that Auntie always used cream when she was cooking all her veggies, making them taste just a little bit better. But she had a little secret. She never ate any of those cream-infused veggies herself.

Salt: Here I want to talk about salt and the first area of discussion is that the Cargill company of Wayzata, Minnesota (close to Minneapolis) is the biggest supplier of salt to the food industry. And proud of it. This is no secret. From his book, Moss writes from Cargill's own literature. "People love salt. Among the basic tastes—sweet, sour, bitter and salty—salt is one of the hardest ones to live without." And it's no wonder. Salt helps give foods their taste appeal –in everything from bacon, pizza, snack foods to baked goods. We know that people crave salty foods. And it certainly is not hidden in things like chips or crisps as they are called in other countries. Marketers know how to appeal to our sense of snacking with ads that say, "Bet you can't just eat one." It's no secret that snacking is a big deal for the food industry. It generates US$100 billion annually in the US. So, you know how big a deal it must be for Cargill who sells the salt contained in or on most of these snacks. The company can refine and create a salt on request for different foods and especially for the snacking industry.

For instance, Michael Moss himself likes a kosher salt called Diamond Crystal salt. He writes, "Their crystals are quadrilateral pyramids that are hollowed out like miniature cups and they have flat sides to stick better to food. The hollowing out, allows the salt to have maximum contact with the mouth's saliva. The unique shape enables it to dissolve 3 times faster than normal salt. And that means it races to the brain with faster, bigger jolts of salty flavor." And that's what Cargill calls the "flavor burst" according to Moss.

Also, the company creates different grades of salt to meet their customer's needs:

Flake salt for cheese and cured meats;

Special flake salt for crackers and breadsticks;

Fine Flake Improved salt for icings and soups;

Shur-flo Fine Flour Salt with three additives to ensure a constant flow and to prevent factory dust.

Further to this, Moss admits that salt is a miracle worker in processed foods. It makes sugar taste sweeter, adds crunch to crackers and it delays spoilage so products can enjoy a longer shelf-life. And most importantly, it masks the bitter and dull taste that are characteristics of so many processed foodstuffs before salt is added. Without salt, processed food companies cease to exist. In fact, at Cargill's own baking facilities, Moss was given bread to taste that had no salt in it at all. He stated, "We ate. We gagged. The bread tasted like tin." Such is the requirement of salt in the food we eat.

In fact, a few years ago when Bev and I visited Jordan, we were touring around the tourist site of Petra. There is a very narrow gap (passageway) with huge rock cliffs on both sides. It's amazing to see. But this was an ancient trade route to the north and on to Europe. Camel caravans had to pass through there, tariffs had to be paid and they were paid with salt. Salt was valued higher than gold back in those days because of its demand for cooking and preserving purposes.

Have you ever eaten food that hasn't been cooked with salt? It certainly can taste bland. I cook with salt when I barbecue steaks. You know the wonderful flavour of a perfectly cooked medium-rare steak. Yummm!! But a few times in my life I've had steak that was cooked without salt. To me it was a waste of a perfectly great cut of meat. It took me awhile to figure out what was wrong. Why did it taste differently from what came off the barbeque in my own back yard? Eventually, I realized that the bland tasting steak had been cooked without salt. It makes a world of difference. It looks exactly the same but it tastes so much different. I've also eaten porridge cooked without a pinch of salt. It tastes fairly bland. And corn-on-the-cob tastes great covered with a generous helping of butter *and* the correct amount of salt.

That's proof to me that we do need salt in our diet. But the problem is that too much salt in processed food often leads to numerous health problems. If not in the short term, then certainly into the future. From Michael Moss's book I learned that in 2005, a dietary committee from the FDA in the US, set a maximum limit of 2,300 milligrams of sodium per person per day. At the time, young men were consuming twice that amount. The committee knew they wouldn't be popular but they pointed out that, "If people could go only part of the way in reaching the 2,300 mg. goal, by reducing their intake of salt by even half a teaspoon a day, this alone would annually prevent 92,000 heart attacks, 59,000 strokes and 81,000 deaths, saving the country twenty billion dollars in health-care and other costs." Certainly, this would be a worthwhile endeavour.

Even prior to that, in 2003, in Britain, there was a legislated goal to reduce the amount of salt consumed in that country. In the first six years of the program, the average person's intake of salt fell by 15 percent and the officials hoped for more. At the time, a professor of cardiovascular medicine in London, Graham MacGregor stated, "It has saved the country 10,000 deaths a year from strokes and heart disease through a public health policy that cost virtually nothing." So that's solid evidence that government controls can work when there's a strong will to make it happen. And an interesting side-bar to this is that British travellers to other countries reported that food in other destinations "tasted too salty."

In the book *Salt, Sugar, Fat* there are pages and pages about the ways that companies manipulate these three ingredients to appeal to the taste buds of consumers. Reading it is a virtual eye-opener. But the one that jumps out concerns the snacking industry. Because snacks are such high revenue generators, manufacturers of these products do everything they can to appeal to consumers' tastes and to maintain market share. And to quote again from the book, "Potato chips are not the poster child for junk food, they are the epitome of processed food generally, which use salt, sugar, and fat, sometimes interchangeably to maximize their appeal to consumers. Frito-Lay could take all the salt out of its chips it wanted, to create whatever aura of health it wanted. As long as the chips remain alluring—through their fat, their crunch, their salty flavour from salt substitutes—and the marketing campaigns give you psychological permission to eat as many as you like, they will continue to deliver calories. And that, after all, is the ultimate cause of obesity."

And there is a sad commentary in the book about the numbers of obese people in the US (upward of 200,000) who annually go for gastric bypass surgery to shrink their stomachs to help them cut back on eating. Some of these patients are as young as nine years old. But when they return home from the hospitals, their old cravings are still there. And, according to Moss, "Even under the best circumstances, these patients struggle to get enough of the nutrients we need to survive."

So, having said all this, it's important that you have all the information you need to eat healthily. Learn to read labels and pay attention to what the labels tell you about the portion size and the number of calories in that portion size. We'll talk about a couple of my weaknesses in a later chapter but I want to give you an example here. I buy a 1.5-kg bag of chocolate-covered almonds or a similar size of chocolate covered and candy-coated M&M's. I have them around and when the bag is open, I can eat whatever I want when I want. But I try to limit myself to a few a day. However, when I checked the label, I saw that there are 220 calories in only nine pieces of the chocolate covered almonds. Just nine. So, if you eat only eighteen of them, then you've consumed 440 calories which is a big bite into your 2,000 calories for the day. However, we do have choices and for a long and active lifestyle it's important to make the right ones. For sure, the snack industry doesn't have your best interests at heart. They are most interested in the profits they make from people's habits. Habits that they've helped to create.

The last word about this comes from Michael Moss's book. When you walk through the aisles of grocery stores, you see all the packaging, the colours and the displays that are designed to attract your attention. You must admit it's all so mesmerizing.

Moss states, "You can see the formulas, the psychology, and the marketing that compels us to toss (all these different) items into the shopping cart. They may have salt, sugar, and fat on their side, but we, ultimately, have the power to make choices. After all, we decide what to buy. We decide how much to eat."

Food manufacturers know all about how the food they offer for sale tastes, and Moss found out why the combinations of salt, sugar, and fat are so important. He tasted different foods in various labs and without the bliss point the lab chemists provided, the food often tasted just like he was eating cardboard. But with the proper combinations, they tasted good. And another point is that many of the executives of these companies eat a well-balanced diet of healthy food at home and never touch the stuff they're pushing out the door and profiting from. That makes a lot of sense at least on one level, I guess.

We know that active lifestyles often dictate that we all have to eat meals we don't prepare ourselves. And let's face it, a good meal at a restaurant is quite enjoyable especially if you are enjoying the experience with family or friends. But the upshot of eating foods you don't prepare yourself is to be aware of what is going into your body and be prepared to cut back if you are exceeding your daily maximums of salt, sugar or fat. Processed food is attractive and does taste good (the chemists in the labs have made sure of that) but eating too much of them on a regular basis will undoubtedly show up on the scale and later on with inherent health issues like we've talked about before.

But remember, the three renegades of the processed food industry are only renegades when there is too much of one or the other or all three of them in the food we eat. All three are necessary for our existence. And as I previously mentioned, what would my favourite vegetable, corn-on-the-cob, be like without a generous slathering of butter and coated with just the right amount of salt? (Mmm, delicious!) Anyway, it's up to each one of us to be aware of what we are taking into our bodies and try our best to stay healthy by consuming only what our bodies need. Read the labels and do your best. You can do it! I know you can.

Remember, the three renegades of the processed food industry are only renegades when there is too much of one or the other or all three of them in the food we eat.

TIPS FROM CHAPTER 14:

1. Be aware of the levels of salt, sugar, and fat.

2. Be calorie smart.

3. Processed food does taste good. But why?

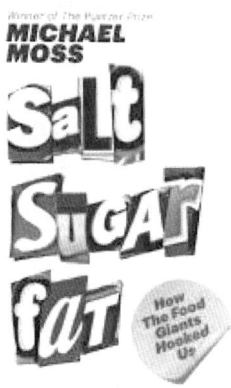

CHAPTER 15

Benefits of a Dog

I considered calling this chapter, *the benefits of pets,* until I thought about it and realized that a cat doesn't really want to go out for a walk in -35C weather. Iguanas aren't very dynamic in getting you up off the couch either. So, I decided to zero in and concentrate on how dogs can affect a person's lifestyle. Since I've been around and owned dogs most of my life, I can vouch for how much our dog Coco gets Bev and me out the door (in all seasons) and assists us with our overall health and well-being.

I love dogs and I'm aware that dogs are attracted to me as well. I tried to come up with an explanation as to why that is and the best idea I can conjure up, is that I was born in the Year of the Dog, on the Chinese calendar. If my sign is the dog, then it makes sense that we would have a natural affinity for each other. And it seems to be true. I get along with most dogs and am not too afraid when approached by a grumpy mean dog. There are some breeds that I would never own, but dog ownership is a matter of choice. We all have our favourites and if a dog meets your needs and you treat it right, then it doesn't matter what breed it is. There's an old saying that goes like this, "try to be the type of person that your dog thinks you are." Your dog loves you unconditionally and as long as you treat it right, then the love you show it will be returned ten-fold. My brother Karl gave me a fridge magnet that reads, "Surround yourself with animals and people who are kind to them." It's so true, we meet some wonderful people when we're out walking our respective dogs.

Loving a dog has many rewards. We'll cover off all the benefits of owning a dog throughout this chapter but for now, I think that many people are aware that a dog can affect their physical, mental and emotional well-being. There are many studies that prove the validity of these statements and we'll address them all later.

When you own a dog, it doesn't take long to learn who is in charge and it isn't always you. But when you're training a puppy there are many things to know. And one of the first things is that dogs want to please their owners, when you make *firm* commands, you show your pup that you mean it. You don't want them to cross the road (for instance) and possibly get run over, so you teach it through firm commands to be obedient. And of course, over time you develop a relationship with your dog and a mutual respect is cultivated. They learn your daily habits and you learn theirs. Dogs are creatures of habit and routine and I want to share a situation that at first just overwhelmed and surprised me until I had the "creatures-of-habit and routine" information explained to me.

One night a few years ago, Bev and I were in bed and we thought our springer spaniel, Coco had settled down, as well. Then she started to bark. It was a different bark than we were used to but it was persistent. Dogs have different barks for different reasons. This time we knew the mail person wasn't delivering mail, it also wasn't the strong "Get away, this is my yard" bark when other dogs are encroaching on our lawn. And it wasn't the "someone is coming up the driveway," bark either. This one had a different tone to it and finally I went to check. There was Coco on the landing looking at the front door and telling me that I had not turned the latch on the deadbolt of the door. Now, this is something I do every night and she knows it. So, when I didn't do it this one night, she was sharp enough to let me know in the only way she knew how.

And there are many stories of people awakened by their dog after their house caught fire. Many folks would have perished from smoke and fire if their dogs weren't around to alert them.

I've always felt that dogs are good for kids in the house. A dog is loyal of course and lavishes unconditional love. Children soon learn that a dog is a living breathing animal who cares for them and will listen to anything they have to say to it. They can have a one-on-one conversation with the dog about whatever is going well or not-so-well for them on a particular day. My four girls grew up with a dog their whole lives and they all love dogs to this day. Dogs teach children responsibility of pet ownership, it teaches them compassion and I've even heard that children who grow up with a dog in their life, tend to be more intelligent. I'm not sure about that last statement but I do know that having a dog around helps with a child's self-esteem and their confidence in dealing with other people. I'm not even sure how that works, but I've seen it in my own household over the years.

We've mentioned it earlier, but dogs get their owners up and going. Springer spaniels are very active dogs. As a pup and a young adolescent dog they want to please and they also love to run. Off leash, they run and run and run. They're loyal to family so they don't generally run away. But they are so much fun to watch as they run and romp and sniff and smell, all the while keeping one eye on where exactly you are. But they need their exercise and if you take them for a walk/run twice a day, they'll catch onto the routine pretty darn fast and will expect you to be *ready to go* at that particular time of day. What that means is they get you up and going. And of course, responsible pet owners will get up off the couch and take their dog out for a walk. And that includes through every season and all types of weather. We find it very interesting as we meet the die-hard walkers, runners and dog owners out in all kinds of weather either in summer or winter.

But the not so dedicated owners tend to be fair-weather dog walkers. One lady we met on the trail for the first time this past spring was walking her dog and said, "It sure is nice to be able to get out and walk the dog again for a change." This was after a normal winter

(2020-2021) but there had been a few very cold days. We hadn't seen them all winter and for sure not when it was -35 Celsius. I just don't know what that poor dog did for exercise all winter. It possibly just wandered around a living room or was sent out to the back yard to get its own exercise and do its business. I don't believe that a dog that is treated that way, gets enough required exercise. Or what about the people who exercise their dog by driving their car while the dog runs along beside. The dogs get their exercise—but what about their owners?

There really is no excuse for not getting out in cold weather. Today's clothing is lightweight and definitely made to keep us warm even on the coldest days. If you're a senior reading this book, then you'll know how poorly insulated the winter clothing used to be. How heavy it was and awkward to put on. On real cold days, several layers were needed to the point where a person could hardly walk. Sounds a bit like the old story of walking up-hill both ways, five miles to school and back, and eating frozen beet sandwiches for lunch. All jesting aside, there really is no excuse with today's modern clothing to not giving a dog the exercise it needs, even in winter. And speaking of modern clothing, there are booties and coats for dogs as well. I never saw any of that when I was growing up. Pampered puppies, some people might think. And of course, they do have their own fur coats but some breeds don't have much of that to keep them warm in winter. A short walk for even those types of dogs is good for them.

Other benefits of dog ownership keep popping up on the different websites that I visited. One of them is social interaction. It's so true, because if two strangers meet and they both have a dog, there's instantly something to talk about. "What breed is your dog? What is his or her name? How old is your dog? Do you come this way often? Do you live close-by?" There are many more questions and answers but, all of a sudden, you've met and chatted with a complete stranger. And you've gladly exchanged information about each other and your dogs. It's a standing joke about these encounters in that you always remember the name of that little curly black dog you met two weeks ago, but be darned if you can remember the owner's name. And it is the same with them. Eventually, you get around to asking these dog owners their name again.

Better health through dog ownership. A number of studies I read talked about how older adults, even ones up into their eighties who walked a dog, were more fit, had a lower BMI (remember that one, body mass index), had fewer complications from daily living, and didn't need to see their doctor so often. In other words, walking a dog every day helps a person lose unneeded weight or helps them maintain their body weight, especially if they are already at the correct weight for their body size. One study suggested that people lost weight while walking dogs they didn't own. The walkers said they were doing it because the dogs needed to be walked. But who was it benefiting the most?

More than one study pointed out that owning a dog can help lower cholesterol levels, reduce blood pressure levels and lower blood triglyceride levels. As we know, elevated levels of one or all of these can lead to higher risks of a heart event like a heart attack. And further studies showed that a person who has a dog companion has a higher survival rate after a heart event. I believe that this is another good reason to own a dog. But of course, I'm biased about that. Can you tell?

Dogs can help reduce stress. I saw with my own eyes how a therapy dog helped a person who had been severely traumatized, to study and learn and obtain high marks just by its presence in the classroom. Something that wouldn't have been possible without the dog being nearby. There is a solid physical reason for the existence of therapy dogs and a lot of it centres around the need to relieve stress in a person's life. Therapy dogs can help ease depression of people from all walks of life and from all age groups, but especially for people who are sick. It's no accident that we see dog visitations on different wards in hospitals or in nursing homes.

Dogs also have been known to heal rifts in dysfunctional families and failing marriages.

As people get older (as we all do), dogs can help to fill a void in their lives. Many folks who have lost a loved one find solace in the companionship of a dog. The dog gives them something to do on a daily basis, like the responsibility of feeding and walking it. Getting out is important and we've already discussed the benefits of exercise folks get when they are out with their furry companions. To say nothing about the dog getting an owner out of bed in the morning. And I've read that pet owners over the age of 65, visit their doctor around 30 percent fewer times than non-pet owners do. Although other pets were helpful in this regard, dog ownership demonstrated the best results.

You may have heard about a dog's ability to detect certain diseases. I don't know a lot about this but I've been told that some dogs are trained to sniff out certain cancers like bladder cancer, prostate cancer, and kidney or skin cancers. Some dogs have even been trained to detect Covid 19. Now those would be highly trained dogs, but there are anecdotal stories about household dogs sensing that something wrong is happening with their owner's body and alerting the household. A few people who got treatment for their ailments were super grateful to their dogs for alerting them or someone else to their previously undetected health problems.

You've no doubt heard about recent information on peanut allergies that shows how exposing infants to peanut butter after six months of age and beyond can help prevent peanut allergies later on. Well, guess what? New research has shown that having pets in the house around newborns and for their first year of life can actually reduce the chance of them developing allergies. This goes against the 1990s' wisdom of the day, that claimed that pets were responsible for the increase of children's allergies. So, grandparents, don't worry about your new grandchild being around the family pet. It's not a problem it was once thought to be. Another good bonus to dog ownership.

We recently had our dog Coco at the vet clinic for her up-to-date rabies shot. The young vet was concerned that her weight was up a bit from the last time. She would like to see a drop of two to four pounds. So, what to do? If the dog were younger, she would have said, "Try to exercise her a bit more." That's easy to do with an active springer. All you do is take them out for an extra run every day. They would love that and it would probably do the job. But with a twelve-year-old dog who is slowing down from arthritis and a cruciate ligament problem, the other obvious choice is to cut down on the amount we give her to eat. Aha! *Reduce portion size*, one of the major keys in my weight-loss program. If it works for me, it should work for our dog so we cut back a bit at each feeding and at our last visit our vet was pleased to see that Coco had lost 8 pounds.

The lesson is that older dogs, like older people don't need as much daily food as they used to. They just aren't as active. So, if the answer for an older dog to lose weight is to cut back on the amount of food it gets, then doesn't it make sense that the same answer should apply to humans as well?

I know there are folks who are reading this who will say, "I've never owned a dog and now you're telling me that if I want to get in shape, I need to get myself a dog!" Or it might be that you live in a condo or apartment where dogs aren't allowed. I'm not suggesting that everyone go out and get a dog. No, indeed not! I'm just pointing out that dogs can help with a person's overall well-being. But I believe that everyone could try to become a little more mobile. Perhaps, your condo or apartment block has a gym room you could use. Maybe there's a fitness instructor who comes around every week. Take advantage of these opportunities if you have a real desire to shed some weight. If none of these ideas will work for you, perhaps you could invest in a stationary bicycle or treadmill. Some of these items are available at discount prices by their owners and often they are hardly used. The means to get active is available. It's up to you to decide if you want to get moving or not. A dog in your life can help get you motivated.

I'd like to end this chapter with another quote from Dr. Richard Blouw, who suggests, *"Start with baby steps, get a friend, dog or relative involved, and keep going. Get off the bus a few blocks before home or work, take the stairs instead of the elevator, walk to the corner store to get a few things rather than taking the car, plan holidays that involve activities of a physical nature, join a group or club that does an activity you'd like to learn, and good things will happen."*

Many people are aware that a dog can affect people's physical, mental and emotional well-being.

TIPS FOR CHAPTER 15:

1. Dogs are loving loyal companions.

2. Dogs get you up and going.

3. More fresh air and exercise are benefits of dog ownership.

LARRY GOMPF

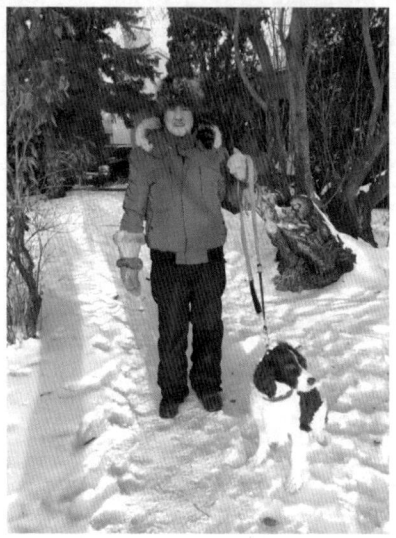

Me with Coco on a cold day

CHAPTER 16
How Fit is the Retired Farmer?

I was going to start out by naming this chapter *Sex and the Retired Farmer* but then I thought that readers might think I was using it only to grab their attention. Mainly because we all know that that word (sex) sells copy all the time. I really wanted to use that title to draw attention to something that I have been observing (along with seeing my own profile) for many years now. And that is a burgeoning waistline amongst middle-aged and older farmers as they near retirement and have slowed down their physical activity.

And for city folks reading this book, you could substitute the name farmer for contractor, semi-driver, or office-worker, because I also see the same phenomena there as well. But because I've been closest to the farming community over my lifetime, I chose to pick on farmers and draw attention to what I'm seeing. And I'm not doing this to be mean or to mock anyone. I just hope that by explaining my observations, I might help out some families in the future. How? Well, if this book convinces just a few folks to change their long-ingrained habits, then maybe, just maybe, a few of them might be able to share more healthy and happy years with their loved ones. That's my true desire for this book.

So, if this chapter isn't about sex, then what is it about? Really, it's about technology and how that has been a labour-saver over so many generations. My generation remembers what it was like to farm without a lot of mechanization. We were mechanized somewhat, but I remember watching guys stooking and pitching sheaves. All those farmers and their helpers were lean and wiry. Not an ounce of fat anywhere to be found. That was a result of many long days of hard manual labour.

I myself had the wonderful experience of mowing and raking with horses. And I hated it! They never seemed to want to do what I wanted them to. They always seemed to want to reach down and get a mouthful of hay as I tried to keep them going straight, even when they had on a muzzle that was supposed to stop them from doing that. Or they would be switching their tails and just about hit me in the face, or they might noisily pass the most putrid smelling gas that you can imagine. Right into my face! Or one time when I saw a bee land on the rump of one horse and I said to myself, "Horse, whatever you do, don't switch your tail at that bee or

I'm going to get it!" You know what happened next, right? Sure enough, the horse switched and that bee came right back and stung me on the neck. I was so mad at that horse and my neck hurt so bad, that I almost quit raking that day. But I didn't. My brother Garnet loved all that work with horses but I could never understand why.

But I digress. The point I'm making about *back in the day* was that the work was physically demanding and most farmers never put on an ounce of fat no matter what they ate or how much. Everyone was the same. Whether they pitched bales all day, stacked hay, shovelled grain, forked manure, or dug post holes by hand, a farmer worked physically hard every day. He earned every bite of food he ate.

Now, fast-forward to today. Technology has been every farmer's boon but it has also made him a victim of the table. It's great to go out every day and lift and move bales with the front-end loader. Or move a grain auger around using the hydraulics on the tractor. I can name hundreds of labour-saving devices that have made farming easier from a physical standpoint. Heck, with auto-steer installed in the cabs, the operator doesn't even have to steer the tractor, the combine or the sprayer as it moves down the field. Those of us who notice, just love looking at those straight lines down the field as a result of GPS technology. Now I'm not naïve enough to believe that every farmer has all this labour-saving equipment. However, I think it's great that farmers get to use this available technology. But one of the main drawbacks is that farmers are not as physically active as they used to be. And that round of golf once a week with a steak and a pop or beer doesn't really compensate. We have to face the fact that farmers generally are not putting in the number of hard-working hours that they once did. And as they approach retirement, it shows.

I wrote this chapter in particular to show the pitfalls of eating too much while doing less physical work. I'm not pointing fingers, but I know that farmers can be a most stubborn group and they have a lot of pride. Even though their good wife (who is always a great cook) tries to get her man to ease up on his eating ways, old habits die hard. If you've always had breakfast with two or three eggs, three or four strips of bacon or sausage, and toast and jam and coffee with sugar, then why not continue? Same with a big lunch or dinner and an afternoon snack and/or a bedtime snack. Why should it be any different now?

It's because the technology we've just been bragging about means most farmers really don't need to consume as much food as they used to. Driving around in the half-ton after eating a normal big breakfast is a lot different than when a farmer would be on a skid piling bales all morning. If a person still eats like he did back in those days, then it's little wonder I see what I do at farm shows. Many folks these days are wearing suspenders just like our grandfathers used to. It's not because they are making a fashion statement. No, it's because suspenders make it easier to carry around the extra weight that's around the belly. Guys just aren't as fit as they used to be. Strong, yes, but not necessarily fit. There is a difference.

Rural communities are simply what they are. Everyone is friendly and willing to help out. That's why if neighbours see their friends out walking, they'll always stop and ask if they need a ride somewhere. The assumption often is that there's a breakdown and that the neighbour could use a lift home. And because everyone knows what a person is doing (or should be doing), then someone out walking while swinging their arms or twisting their torso to get more physical exercise is often snickered at behind their backs. That's just the way it is. Nothing wrong with it, that's just common practice in rural communities.

Maybe young farmers go to gyms or have their own gym room set up in their house, but a farmer who is nearing retirement might be teased if he were to tell his fellow coffee-shop patrons that he was going to join a gym and try to get a little more fit. Peer pressure often keeps a guy away. But it shouldn't. Think about living a healthier lifestyle and being around for a longer time to spend with your family. My wife Bev and I can only imagine the shape we'd be in now if we hadn't joined Sharon Couldwell's great fitness class seventeen years ago. We are pretty sure we wouldn't be as active as we are. I suggest to everyone reading this book that it's never too late to start shedding a few pounds and become more fit. It just takes a strong desire to do so. And you can start anytime. Start by eating less at tomorrow's meal and getting up and going for a walk. Those are a couple of the things you need to do to start you on your journey to a *slimmer* and healthier you.

Now don't get me wrong, farmers are very strong people. Growing up, although I did farm work all the time, I was never one of those tough farm kids. Almost anyone could beat me at arm wrestling. Many farmers who are ready to retire have a lot of upper body strength. I won't deny that, but when you look at the waistline of many of them, it's easy to see that even though they have a lot of upper body strength, many of them are carrying too much weight around their middle and are just not as fit as they could be.

But why should I care? It's because of what is written in the chapter on diseases like diabetes, heart disease, strokes, and cancer, carrying extra weight can lead to a future disaster. And I *do* want all of you reading this book to get the message to become more fit and to live a longer healthier life.

When we talk about farmers and fitness, remember when we used to walk the fields after the crops germinated and started to grow? That footwork kept us healthier because of the walking we did, often from corner to corner in a field. We were looking for and identifying the weeds so we would know what crop protection product we would have to apply. We were possibly checking for insect damage, but at least we were getting some exercise as we walked, stopped and knelt down to get a close-up look at our fields. It was healthy exercise. But what do we do now?

Now farmers either hire an agrologist to do the scouting, or the local dealer has field scouts who will find out what is in the fields and recommend the best product for the job. Or the farmer might choose to do his own scouting and ride out and around the fields on a quad. That's good, it gets him out and across the fields quickly and any exercise benefits come from getting on and off the machine. But really, it's not like actually walking the field. That's when farmers used to get the greatest health benefits. And they knew each of their fields more intimately.

I know from observation that many of the next generation of farmers are aware that they must do something to stay fit. They understand the benefits of matching farm strength with physical fitness. I'm hoping they carry that understanding through to their retirement, and beyond. Maybe they will. If they live near like-minded folks who also believe in staying fit, perhaps as a group it will work for them. Right now, I want to concentrate on grabbing the attention of their fathers and their grandfathers, and I'm hoping that guys from those two generations will accept the idea that getting and staying fit could be a health benefit that will help them live a longer, healthier life—a life that is free from aches and pains and free from the need for health-care interventions, plus a reduced need for joint replacements or support from prescription drugs. If you think about it, you know that *it is* possible. And it's not just men, I'm afraid to say. Some women could also take this advice to heart. Or anyone of a certain age or occupation.

And once again (at risk of sounding like a broken record), I wouldn't want anyone to lose weight too quickly. Just think of when you last might have been a young, wiry, strong, slim, and dashing young man who all the women were eager to dance with. If you can recall those days, then try to remember how old you were when it started to change. That's right! It wasn't last year or five years ago or ten. Perhaps, it was some twenty-five years ago or more.

What I'm trying to say is that it took a long time to put on the extra weight. If you were fifty and now you are seventy-five, like me, then that is twenty-five years of slowly gaining weight. And like me, the extra weight probably slipped up on you and you weren't even aware it was happening. So, if you are keen on shedding the extra belly fat (visceral fat) you're now carrying, then please work at getting rid of it slowly. I'm proof that the slow method does work. So here is what I want you to do.

In the privacy of your bedroom, in your underwear, look at your sideways profile in a mirror. If you are happy with what you see, then maybe you don't even need to finish reading this book. But if you see a pronounced "pot belly" or what is commonly called a "beer belly" then maybe you'd like to start to get rid of it slowly. Gone should be the days when you proclaim to the world, "This thing took a while but here it is all bought and paid for!" Or, "This ole belly got here one beer at a time." Sorry folks, that extra weight should no longer be a topic of humour. I'm not laughing about it and maybe you shouldn't either. In the future, along with that 'good old belly', could be lurking a fatal health event just waiting to happen. And that's why I'm not laughing. Neither you nor your family should want that to occur. It's your choice and I'll say it again, you can lose weight even by eating everything you've ever eaten. Just slow up on the amount you're eating, pay attention to your weight trends and become more mobile. It's easy to start today.

Now, remember when I said that I was tempted to name this chapter, "Sex and the retired farmer!!" I was joking at the time, but I've thought about this for a while. Nature plays a little trick on us as we grow older. The close physical desire we once had for each other tends to slow down along with the libido. That's normal. But the level of sexual attraction also slows down faster when people are overweight. It's no longer, "Not tonight, honey, I have a headache!"

It's more like, "I just don't seem to be interested anymore." And often the comeback is, "I'm not really that interested, either." Sigh!! That becomes the pattern and libido seems to wane at far too early a stage in life. And it's partly because of one or the other or both partners are carrying extra weight they don't need. But what *might* happen if both of you were able to get down to what is considered a natural body weight for your body size? It could be possible that the "sparks" might fly again with renewed intensity. I guess you'll never know unless you set a target to accomplish that goal. But maybe everything is fine in that department even while you are carrying more weight. Congratulations to you, but my assumption is that it would be the exception rather than the rule.

On page ninety-seven of a wee book, that I picked up at a garage sale, called *Meditations from The Road* by M. Scott Peck, the following was written. "Couples sooner or later always fall out of love, and it is at the moment when the mating instinct has run its course that the opportunity for genuine love begins."

Think about that statement! The romantic love people initially have for each other can wane fairly quickly after the marriage vows, but solid and genuine love lasts for a lifetime for couples who work at the relationship and for couples who are truly meant for each other. But introducing a bit of the old "spark" wouldn't hurt the relationship either. So, get up off the couch, the half-ton seat, the tractor seat, the combine seat, the front-end loader seat or any seat, and work hard to surprise yourself and your spouse. There is still lots of fun to be had in life.

And wouldn't it be great in a few years to have your friends, relatives and neighbours say, "Boy you're looking good. What diet did you go on?" Especially if you've never told them that you were going to slow down your eating habits and that you were planning to become more active. The choice is yours. Go for it. Carpe diem! And good luck!

It's never too late to start shedding a few pounds and become more fit. It just takes the strong desire to do so. And you can start anytime.

TIPS FROM CHAPTER 16:

1. Farmers aren't as active as they used to be.

2. GPS has helped rural folks be less active.

3. Learn to eat less and exercise more.

LARRY GOMPF

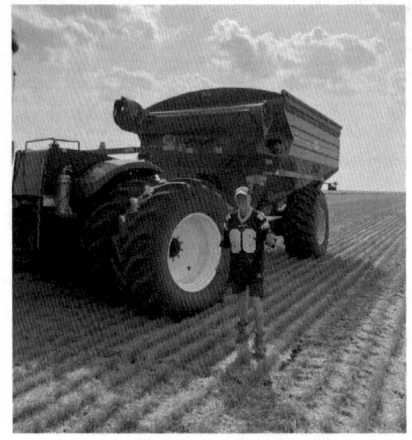
Beside the grain cart

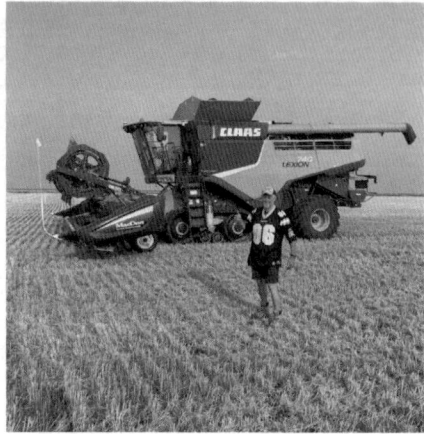
In front of the combine

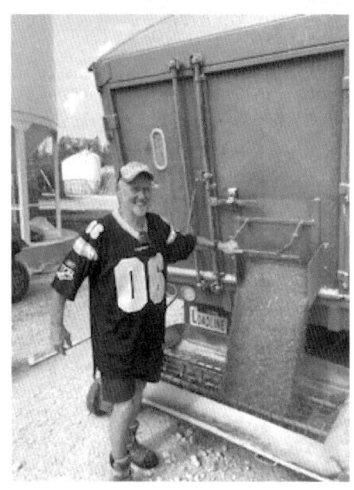
Unloading wheat - harvest 2021

CHAPTER 17
Living For Your Grandkids

You've probably all seen the bumper sticker that reads something like this: "If I'd known that grandchildren would be so much fun, I'd have had them first." It's not written to discount your own children but it really is the essence of grandparenting. Grandchildren can be so much fun. Their innocence, their cute sayings, the fact they are always listening when you talk, their sense of humour, their eager willingness to learn and accept what you have to offer, all make being around grandchildren such a great experience. Most grandparents would say that there are no greater times, than the times they spend with their grandchildren.

So why would I write about grandchildren in a book about losing weight and keeping it off? It's simply because I'm hoping that because of the grandkids (and for some folks, great-grandkids), you'll want to be around to enjoy them. And you know they want you to be around to play with them, teach them games, teach them life skills and mentor them as they make their way through life. If you're healthy and fit, it's so much better and super rewarding. You'll be a continuing part of their life and you'll contribute so much more to their overall experience if you are an active participant in their life. A healthy grandparent is a lot more fun.

When I was a little boy of about four or five, I remember my Uncle Eldon Walton coming from Alberta to visit us on the farm. Out of the blue, he got down on the floor and rolled a ball back and forth to me and we laughed and had a good time. It was the first time an adult had ever done that and you can see the impact it had on me. It was fun and I never forgot it. But think about that for a second. To children, adults look huge. Big and tall and towering way above the height of a toddler. They always have to look up, way up. Then think about how it must feel to have a big, tall adult (parent, aunt, uncle, or grandparent) come down to their level on the floor. All of a sudden, you are in their space and they love it that you are there.

After that experience with my uncle, I vowed that I would get on the floor at my children's level and play with them whenever I got a chance. In other words, I wanted to be the big kid to them. And most recently, with my then four-year-old grandson, Simon, and his two-year-old sister, Halle, we played hide-and-go-seek. They loved it and there was lots of laughter as one or the other discovered the others or were discovered. Is there more fun than unsolicited childhood laughter? During those times of hiding and then being found, I squeezed myself into some very tight and narrow spaces. That's the most fun when you can do that and they are baffled as they run around looking for you. Those are special moments that some people just miss out on, especially if they're too overweight or lack the mobility to move around in tight corners like that. To me, that's what grandparenting is all about.

Something I learned recently, is that if a child starts to stutter (and their speech is disrupted by repetitions or long pauses) at an age when they are learning to speak (two to five years old), it's a good idea for you to demonstrate that they have your undivided attention when talking to them. Look them in the eye and talk to them at their face level. This worked for the son of my book-coach and I was curious to learn more about it, so I called my sister-in-law, Monica Gompf, who is a retired speech and language pathologist, and she gave me some important information about how this works.

Monica says that stuttering may occur when a child's speech/language development hasn't yet advanced enough for them to be able to properly express what they want to say. In other words, they have not developed a large enough vocabulary and command of our complex language to formulate the information they wish to express. "They try to fit sentences together and may demonstrate hesitations, repetition of words or sounds or phrases as they try to express their ideas," she says. Young children hear their parents talking and they understand the language, but they struggle with the complex expressions that their parents can articulate with ease. "Their language command just isn't there yet," she adds.

Monica went on to say that one of the techniques recommended for parents is to look at the child and be at eye level with them so they feel they have your attention. "Having eye contact by being at their level, not correcting or interrupting them, and speaking more slowly to the child, is a model that helps them to slow down as they work though the formulation and expression of their message."

And that is exactly what helped my then-four-year-old grandson Simon get over his wee stuttering problem. My daughter Jenny says Simon no longer stutters. He eventually outgrew it.

Now I want to tell you about the fishing wall of fame at our cabin at Eagle Lake in northwest Ontario. As each child catches their first fish on the lake, they end up with an eight-by-ten picture of themselves, with a mile-wide grin on their face, as they hold up their catch of the day. The oldest grandchild is Josh, who is now twenty-two. His first Northern pike was caught on his sixth birthday with his brand-new rod and reel outfit. His brother Ajay (now eighteen) caught a smallish walleye when he was five years old. And you should have seen him smile and cheer when he pulled in a thirty-six-inch Muskie on a single-hook pickerel jig when he was thirteen years old.

Xavier (now twelve) caught his first (a pike) when he was six years old. We took Savannah who was six, and Ramone, who was four, fishing on July 1, of 2018. After some time when the kids were starting to get bored, Ramone snagged and landed a small perch. But it might as well have been a fifty-pound Muskie, he was so excited. After a while his sister said, "I'm never going to catch a fish!" So, I told her that no, she should say, "I am going to catch a fish!"

So, she stated, "I am going to catch a fish," and within two minutes, she pulled in a beautiful eighteen-inch walleye. She also was excited but the best part was when their father Steve said, "I don't know who was more excited, the kids or the grandfather." And it was true. In about one hour we had created two fisher-people. And guess what they both wanted for their upcoming birthdays. That's right, their very own rod and reel and tackle box. Which they got. And, that folks, is what grandparenting is all about. Being there to enjoy those special moments.

Back in late winter in 2021, I got a cell phone after being without one for a very long time. I was having trouble getting up to speed with it and we were also having some issues with our desk-top computer and my wife Bev's phone. We'd go to the MTS service centre and think we'd have all the problems solved, but there always seemed to be a glitch. After a number of times, we finally got everything straightened out but not without a certain level of frustration. (Has that ever happened to you?) Throughout the process, we entered a number of passwords that didn't seem to be working. Later, at my daughter Jenny's house I was explaining to her about "all these passwords that were running around." We looked at then four-year-old Simon and we could tell he was perplexed, so we asked him what was the matter. It turned out that his little mind was trying to visualise all these passwords running around on the table or wherever. When we all realized it, we had a magical moment of enjoying a good laugh as we tried to explain what Grandpa Larry had meant. You have to agree that grandparenting can be a lot of fun. It's so much fun to be a part of those kids growing years.

What is the easiest thing to do with grandchildren? And something that is a lot of fun and rewarding, too? It's simply sitting on a chair, a couch, a recliner, or a bed (or anywhere, for that matter), and reading their favourite book to them. They need a lap and of course that's a warm, safe place for them to be. If you get them to notice pictures on the page, and if you put emphasis on the words as you read, this exercise can be a heck of a lot of fun. And when you ask them what they see on the page, it often is different than what you see on the page. Reading to grandchildren and getting them to read to you is so rewarding. It helps prepare them with their future reading skills. Often, having been read to, results in the successful development of young minds as the kids grow up and make their way in the world.

And I believe that interacting with children as an adult is so important for their development. Remember my uncle who got down on the floor with me. It was such a simple gesture but one that I never forgot. And I think all interactions with children are so very important. We have friends, Neil and Dorothy Strachan at Carman, Manitoba, who have laying hens and Bev's sister Wanda and husband Mike also have a hen house on their acreage at Merrickville, Ontario, south of Ottawa. It's so exciting for their grandchildren to go to Grandma and Grandpa's place to collect eggs and to watch and to listen to the peaceful clucking of the hens or hear the rooster crow, if there is one. What a wonderful learning process it is for everyone involved!

During Christmas holidays in 2019, we went to southern Ontario at Collingwood to be with our family who had recently moved there. Dad, Jesse, and Mum, Michelle (daughter) welcomed us to their place and we had a marvelous time with their family, Aven (eight at the time), JJ (who was six), and Raine (who was three). We went tobogganing, made snowmen, helped make cookies, played floor hockey a lot, and of course had a blast watching those kids open their Christmas presents. When we were building a snowman, the snow was great for rolling up, so our snowman just kept getting bigger and bigger. Even wee Raine was bringing rolled up snow for the creation of even a bigger snowman. And of course, we were able to read to them in person. They've grown older, but the recent past with Covid has limited visiting with any of our grandchildren, so isn't it great to have Facetime and Zoom available so the kids don't forget. These connections helped out during that restrictive time and we were grateful for that.

It's all these types of experiences that keep young people coming back to visit their grandparents and each time the experiences are different as they grow up in those environments. There's important relationship-building going on that you'd be hard pressed to put a monetary value on. It's priceless and is ever so meaningful. And it keeps happening over and over again. And as grandparent, it's so much fun to attend birthday parties and see the reactions of the young ones as they get to unwrap a gift of something they have been wanting. The pictures again are priceless. And each time is so different as you watch them grow up over the years.

I have to share this little story about our grandson Xavier, who is twelve, and his sister, Savannah who is ten. When Xavier was one year old, after "Happy Birthday" had been sung to him, he was presented with a piece of chocolate cake on the tray of his high-chair. No one was ready with a camera so when Xavier dug in with both hands and proceeded to cover his whole face with cake, the Kodak moment was lost. Two years later, when his sister was celebrating her first birthday, everyone was ready with a camera to take all kinds of pictures. But Savannah disappointed us by daintily reaching out and taking a wee bit of cake in her fingers and putting it in her mouth all clean and tidy. Why am I telling you this? These stories are what grandparenting is all about. Memories are created that last forever.

Raising a child is a responsibility for everyone involved in that child's life. You've heard the expression, "It takes a village to raise a child." It's so true and think about your own role in helping to raise your grandchildren. You are so much a part of their life and without being demanding, you can mentor them and teach them skills that you've learned over your lifetime. Skills like baking and decorating cookies and cakes, how to sew on a button or how to build things or how to repair car engines or lawn mowers. It's all a part of their training to be good citizens of the world. And you don't necessarily have to be a grandparent. Kids have lots of great experiences with favourite aunts and uncles as well.

But it's so important for grandparents to know and understand their roles in raising their grandchildren. It goes way beyond just filling them full of sweets and sending them home to their parents. When grandparents are in good physical shape (i.e., in good health), then the odds are they'll get to enjoy their grandchildren for a long time. Not only that, their grandchildren will be able to count on having their grandparents around for a longer time as well. Grandparents who will continue to mentor, teach and love them unconditionally.

a slimmer you

Doesn't thinking about that make you want to be in your best physical shape for the future? A future that includes your grandchildren. It's your choice!

When two of my grandchildren caught their first fish within minutes of each other, their father Steve said, "I don't know who was more excited, the kids or their grandfather."

TIPS FROM CHAPTER 17:

1. Grandparenting is very rewarding.

2. Being fit keeps grandparents active.

3. Mentoring grandchildren is an important role.

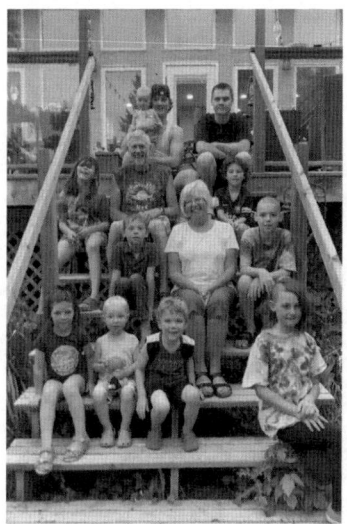

Bev and me with our 11 eleven grandchildren- July 2021

CHAPTER 18
Living to be 110

Why do you suppose that some people live to 110 years old and are still active right up to the end? Most of us might answer, "Because they have strong inherited genes." And that answer might be the key to some of the great results. Or, we might think that these centenarians (plus) were just plain lucky, or that they were better able to fight off the communicable diseases that are always around. Again, that might be a valid answer or at least a part of it. But I think that a good part of the answer lies in attitude. Did the person live his or her life always with a glass half empty or a glass half full? The answer to that question might be an important key.

We know that everyone faces stress and adversities in life. How centenarians handled those set-backs might be the secret to their longevity. Did they wilt under the pressures or did they face up to the tough challenges and come out the other side better and stronger and more able to take on the world? You know the saying that when life gives you lemons, you make lemonade. I'd bet that most folks over 100 years of age clung to that philosophy. The main thing is they didn't give up.

One time I got a chance to visit a man who lived in my mother-in-law's assisted living place. He told me a scary story about being captured in World War II by the Germans during a D-Day mission. He and his fellow regiment burst their way into German occupied French territory. They were supposed to have aerial back-up but it never showed up. They were captured and were put into cattle cars, but before they entered, they were given a piece of bread and a small amount of water. They were told to eat small bits and drink very little of the water because it had to last four days. Well, he sadly told me that they were stuck in those rail cars for twenty-eight days. I was in tears as told me his tale. But worse was yet to come. They finally got out of the railcars because someone got through to the commander in charge and told him that if they weren't released from the car, they were all going to die very soon. They got out but ended up in a POW camp and the man in charge was none other than the Butcher of Lyon, Klaus Barbie. The stories that I was told about how these POWs were treated would make your hair stand on end. I don't think he'd ever shared them with anyone before.

Why am I telling you this sad tale? Because this man was the kindest most wonderful man you could ever meet. He was certainly given lemons and made lemonade. He was past 95 when he told me this story and he passed away just before reaching 100 years old. He was one of those wonderful people who focused on the positive in life, was a man of principle and was a ray of sunshine to those around him. People like him never gave up on life, even when experiencing the bleakest of times. His determination is a real inspiration to those of us who don't think we have the inner strength to carry on through much less-trying situations. It's so important to stay focused.

And remember Jackrabbit Johannsen? One of my inspirations for writing this book. He had that type of determination and he helped thousands of young people learn to cross-country ski. Through hard work in setting out and cutting trails in the bush, he made it possible for young people to take up the sport and he taught them how to enjoy it like he did. He never let obstacles stand in his way. He is credited with bringing cross country skiing to Canada. He was instrumental in building many ski trails and ski jumps that are still in use today in Ontario, in the Eastern townships of Quebec, in the Laurentians and in the Adirondack Mountains of New York. The Jackrabbit ski program is still taught to youngsters across Canada in his memory. Jackrabbit lived to 111 years old and he certainly did not let his age hinder his ambitions and goals.

He is definitely a person who can be used as a role model to get up off the couch. And remember it was Jackrabbit Johannsen who said, "I owe my longevity to that fact that I always push back from the table when I feel I could still eat more!"

My own mother-in-law, Jean Jamieson lived to a wonderful age of 99 years and 4 months. She approached life with a super positive attitude and never dwelled on the negatives that life throws at us on a daily basis. She loved to read and tackled historical biographies with a keen sense of curiosity. Although her eyesight was failing her and she couldn't sustain reading for long periods of time, in her last year she managed to make her way through books of interest that were many pages long. She loved to read biographies of the Royal family and others. Jean often remarked how glad she was that "I still have all my marbles!" And that's the key, isn't it? Living to a ripe old age with a positive attitude is great if you *still have all your marbles.* One leads to the other. If you've always had a positive attitude to life, maybe you'll live a long life with a strong clear mind.

In those Covid-19 isolation times, of 2020 to 2022, it was never clearer than it's been, that people need interactions with other people in order to live a healthy lifestyle. Letters to personal counsellors in local papers have a daily stream of questions about, "How do I handle my loneliness?" Kids, who used to claim that they hated school, were wishing they could get back to the classroom because they learned better there. Not only that, they were lonely for their classmates. They truly missed the social aspect of school. It's only a small minority of students who truly hate going to school (for whatever reason) who did not want to go back.

And what do we know about people whose whole life was consumed with their job? Many of you know someone who retired from their lifetime position without a real plan about retirement, only to die within a short period of time. It's sad but true. They didn't have anything to replace the job that they'd cherished so much. And they were lost souls. Everyone should have a bucket list of things to accomplish.

When I think about those types of people, I think of the senior farmer Mr. Lodge from Baldur, Manitoba. Back in the 1980s, this man was still farming a small acreage. He had 160 acres and was planting about 80-100 acres every year. His equipment was small and older. I remember a six-foot one-way, an older low horse-powered tractor and a ten or twelve-foot drill. He was in his nineties, and folks would say to him, "Why are you doing this every year when you could be living comfortably here in the manor in town?" And his reply was simple, "If I moved into the manor, I would die shortly after." He was self-aware enough (and probably stubborn as well) to know that the farm gave him a purpose. He always had something to look forward to. He had to plan what he was going to plant, line up seed for the spring, get some fertilizer (if he used any), do the seeding, the spraying and then swath and combine his crop. And then he had to work his land in the fall. It kept him busy until freeze up. In other words, the little farm on which he was living and growing a crop gave him a reason to live. In the manor, he would have lost his purpose for living and he knew it.

In this old fellow's world, there wasn't a lot of socialising happening, but in many older folk's lives, socialisation is what keeps them going. If you ever visit an assisted living complex, you'll see seniors playing cards and other games, gathering for sing-songs and meeting every day before, during and after lunch. In small towns there are senior's centres where folks go to socialize and play cards or work on a puzzle. And think about all the "lies" that are spun daily around a coffee-shop as people gather to share stories about their past glory days. It keeps folks going.

And volunteering locally or at bigger events gives seniors a chance to be involved in the bigger picture. I was a driver at the 1999 Pan American games, at the 2007 Women's World Hockey tournament and at the Roar of the Rings Olympic curling playdowns in 2013 all in Winnipeg. It gave me a purpose and was a lot of fun meeting people from around the country and from around the world. Without the volunteerism of eager seniors, many events would just not happen. At the annual folk festival held at Bird's Hill Provincial Park there are hundreds of volunteers. Many are seniors who were there right at the start in 1974. They love going, helping out, listening to the wonderful music from all around the world and socialising with friends they've made over the years. They get to listen to their favourite folk bands for sure, but that isn't the only reason they volunteer their time. It keeps them totally engaged for a very intense five days or more and they love every minute of it.

When I checked, I found that the value of volunteer work in Canada performed by seniors had an annual economic impact of *$10.9 billion*. This information was taken from Volunteer Canada and was listed in June 2019. The value of the work was estimated at $27/hour, which seems high to me but still, the impact on the country is immense. In other words, there would be fewer programs, concerts, sports events, theatre plays, and shows if it weren't for the thousands of senior volunteers. Either there would be fewer of these events or they would cost a heck of a lot more for each patron to attend.

From the internet, I learned that Volunteer Canada is a registered charity that provides national leadership and expertise on volunteerism in order to increase the participation, quality and diversity of volunteer experiences. And I was surprised to learn its headquarters is in my home city of Winnipeg. I also learned of studies conducted in the US in 2013 which indicate that when older people volunteered their services, no matter in what area, they claimed to have better health, they functioned better in their daily lives, they increased their physical activity, they had lower rates of depression and they tended to live longer than folks who didn't volunteer. In effect, volunteering helped with these folk's overall well-being. If you think about it, I'm sure you'll agree that this all makes sense.

And now I have a skill-testing question for you. The answer is on page **157** of this book, but please don't look there until you've carefully thought about your answer and why you chose that answer. The question is this: In a questionnaire, healthy centenarians were asked that if they had a chance to go back and live their life over again, what age would they choose to go back to and start over? Think about what age that would be for yourself. And again, I want you to do this without peeking. It's a fun little exercise to do. Good luck!

Now at first glance this book *A Slimmer You,* appears to be about losing weight. And it definitely is. But in reality, it's about living a fuller life. It's about getting more out of the years you have left. It is about eating well and exercising your body, your muscles, your brain and in the end improving your overall health. If what I'm writing makes sense to you, and you follow what has worked for me, you'll find that losing weight is a by-product of all that you might achieve. You'll have lost the extra weight and for sure you'll look better and feel better too. Not just physically better but mentally as well. And I also believe you'll be a happier person in the end. Isn't it worth giving it a whirl?

I am lucky enough to be involved in a twenty-year longitudinal study on aging. This study is run out of McMaster University in Hamilton, Ontario. It's called the Canadian Longitudinal Study on Aging (CLSA), and is a national long-term study of more than 50,000 individuals who were between the ages of forty-five and eighty-five when the program started. These participants are to be followed until 2033 or until they die. The aim of the CLSA is to find ways to help us live long and live well and to understand why some people age in a healthy fashion while others do not. The CLSA is a longitudinal design, meaning that it follows people over a long period of time. However, researchers will not wait years before results are generated. Many researchers can apply now to access currently collected data to generate findings that will improve our understanding of why some people age in healthy ways and others do not.

Results from the CLSA will

1. Contribute to identify ways to prevent disease and improve health services;

2. Develop better understanding of the impact of non-medical factors, such as economic prosperity and social changes, on people as they age;

3. Answer questions that are relevant to decision-makers to improve health policy and inform government programs and services;

4. Generate new knowledge on many interrelated biological, clinical, psychosocial and societal factors that influence disease, health and well-being;

5. Develop Canadian research capacity and train future generations of researchers who will use the CLSA data and infrastructure to explore previously unimagined areas of research on aging.

I've been a participant at CLSA for many years now and have had to complete all kinds of tests, which include monitoring weight, body scans, blood tests, breathing tests, standing on one leg, walking a taped line, sitting down and getting up from a chair, cognitive tests, hearing and eye tests, and a number of others. At first, I thought my results would compare me to others of my age and gender. Initially I was disappointed to find out that this was not the case. I learned that the study was to determine how aging affects older people and how diet and exercise can actually help people live longer and healthier lives. Yes! I'm all for that, as you know, and to be a part of a study of 50,000 people that can only help develop plans for the future health of the nation means I'm certainly on board.

Now why is it a goal for people to live a long and healthy life? First of all, a lot of us have a bucket list of things we want to do before we no longer can move. It might be to take an RV trip across Canada to see areas of the country we've only heard about or seen on TV and would like to visit. It could be to go to Tuscany, Italy and visit the small villages and vineyards. Or maybe you'd like to go to the Galapagos Islands to see the hundreds-year-old turtles. Many of us have the time and money to fulfill the dreams on our bucket lists. And there are thousands of things to do and even more dreams about doing them, but if we are overweight and our knees or hips no longer work properly, then the bucket-list disappears quite quickly. And then the only response is "what if?"

Some people don't want to retire at all. In the Saturday May 29, 2021, *Winnipeg Free Press* was a story written by Doug Spiers of a ninety-five-year-old lawyer (Gordon Pullan) who has been practising law for seven decades. When asked when he might retire, his quick answer was, "When I get old." He goes into the office Tuesdays, Thursdays, and Saturdays. And he likes Saturdays because there are fewer people there and he gets more work done.

I have a friend (Les Kletke) who is sixty-five who has developed a business as a book coach. He has helped over 100 people develop and write books. He's the person responsible for helping me pull this book together and get it into your hands today. Is he thinking of retiring? No, he wants to continue his business for at least the next ten years. Because of his positive attitude, his sense of humour, and his interest in life, he'll easily make those ten years and more. I just know it. And guess what, folks? He actually adopted some of the measures outlined in this book to help him stay focused on his future goals. The first one he adopted was to start strengthening his core muscles. And he shared with me that directly because of stronger core muscles, his golf drives last summer were consistently fifteen yards farther than before. That was the *only* thing he had done differently. For you golfers who are reading this, maybe strengthening your core muscles could help improve *your* own golf game. I'm just saying.

This is the first book I've ever written. You might ask why I didn't write sooner. Because I guess it took me this long to actually have something to say. I'm seventy-five now and plan to conduct twenty "A Slimmer You" seminars in the next five years. That is, if anyone might be interested enough to hire me to hear what I have to say about the most natural way to lose weight and how to adopt a moderate form of exercise. And to explain the recommendations I make in this book. Maybe by the time I'm eighty, I'll have had enough of all this or maybe I'll be looking forward to another project. The actress Betty White recently passed away. She was just shy of 100 years old and already had another filming project lined up to shortly follow the one she was working on when she died. She was a remarkable woman with a remarkable attitude to life. She never was one to sit in a rocking chair and watch the world go by.

Anyway, we never know how long we have on this earth, so the best thing is to enjoy every day and indulge in activities that leave you with a grateful, positive outlook on life. I think it's the only way to go. Don't you agree?

Living to a ripe old age with a positive attitude is great if you still have all your marbles.

TIPS FOR CHAPTER 18:

1. A positive attitude challenges adversity.

2. Seniors make a difference as volunteers.

3. The longitudinal study will make a difference.

CHAPTER 19
See Say Safety

You've read the stories about weight loss and how it can lead to a longer, healthier, and less stressful life. But in this chapter, I want to write about how to keep yourself alive longer. This time, it's not about weight loss, but it has a lot to do with driving. Almost everyone reading this book has had a close call. These can be very nerve-wracking and even scary. If you're driving when this happens, you may have to pull over and settle your nerves and calm the shakes before continuing on. I can outline a number of close calls in my life and I'm so thankful that nothing serious happened. The most serious one was in the fall of 2014. I was travelling along at highway speed and just about to slip by a pick-up truck pulling a trailer full of hay bales. The small square ones that often weigh about eighty pounds.

I was near the back of the trailer when a single bale came loose from the middle of the trailer and bounced on the highway in front of me. There was no time to react. I couldn't veer to the right as there were vehicles coming fast in that lane and I was right beside the concrete highway divider on my left. So, I just stood on the brake hard, kept the wheel straight, and wondered if I would be smashed from behind as I knew there were vehicles behind me. When the car stopped and the engine died (I was driving a standard-shift vehicle), I couldn't believe that nothing had happened to me. The driver of the pick-up behind me must have seen the bale fall and bounce in front of me and he was able to stop his truck in time. Because nothing had happened, I decided to get out of the car, go around in front, and remove the bale. I hadn't hit it but it had to be somewhere. Lo and behold, when I went to open the car door there was that bale, fully intact and I could only get the door open about half way. It could have killed me or caused me to be in a crippling accident but it hadn't.

I decided to carry on, so I started the car and drove away and was no worse for the wear. I even caught up to the driver of the truck with the trailer of bales and he was totally oblivious. He didn't even know he'd lost a bale. Because I had an appointment downtown in less than an hour, I had to get home, freshen up and continue on my way. And the strange part of this near-miss is that through the whole thing which must have lasted about thirty seconds, I was able to drive on and was very calm. Why? I can't really answer that question, but I just was.

And that leads me to the purpose of this chapter. It's all about possibly keeping you alive and healthy for years to come. This chapter is about *horizon driving*. Many of you haven't heard about horizon driving, so I'll explain. You've all heard about defensive driving and many of you know what that entails. Some of you may have taken courses on how to do it. Well, horizon driving is the term I learned from an owner/instructor of a safety driving course. Every few years, our company would send us for driver skills training to keep us sharp about the rules of the road. The instructor called her defensive driving course, Horizon Driving. Her best clients were former airplane pilots because they were always scanning the horizon ahead and to the side to be aware of their surroundings. That was of course part of their training and what they always practised in the air. And naturally, they continued to do it on the ground as well.

We were taught to scan a few blocks ahead, not just the car length or two ahead of us. Our instructor had us practise looking for anything coming from our left, or our right and be aware what was coming up behind us. She said that it's important to practise horizon driving all the time and in that way you can avoid possible accidents. Serious crashes that happen because some in-a-hurry folks may run a red light or a stop sign and T-bone you. I know of a number of people who experienced that very thing. It happened to a young neighbour of mine and she lost her career as a border services officer because of her injuries. She loved that job but, sadly, had to give it up. She'd been T-boned by somebody who didn't stop at a stop sign.

Or how about a fellow from SW Manitoba whom I knew and respected. He and his wife were stopped at a stop sign at Highway #83 leading onto Highway #1. He was seventy-five at the time and unfortunately drove out into the path of an oncoming semi-truck and both of them were killed. Had he known about horizon driving he might have lived many more years. Horizon driving to me is looking both ways twice or more just in case. From behind, it may look like you are watching a tennis match, but isn't it worth a couple of extra looks if it might save your life? If you've driven for many years, I know that sometimes you've started to move ahead only to slam on your brakes because a car was right there. A car you hadn't seen at first glance. And you end up thanking your lucky stars that you finally did see that car at the last second. Horizon driving gives you another chance. Learn to practise it.

Just a month before my seventy-fifth birthday, I believe I prevented an accident by being alert when I was driving. I was travelling at highway speed on Highway #1 before Falcon Lake, Manitoba and a semi was behind me in my lane. I noticed that an SUV was starting to pass the semi in the other lane beside him. The vehicle was probably one third of the way down the side of the truck when I noticed the semi start to pull out to pass me. I immediately turned right onto the highway shoulder, the semi driver noticed and pulled back and the SUV kept going. The truck driver waved a thanks of gratitude as he slipped by. He knew that a collision was avoided because I was paying attention. The car was possibly in his blind spot or he just wasn't paying attention. The best part of all, is that no-one got hurt. And all this happened in a split second. These incidents always do.

I taught my girls about the importance of horizon driving and to this date they have never been in an accident. In fact, my youngest daughter Jenny was riding with her mum a number of years ago and they were about to turn right onto a side street, when Jenny noticed a pair of little feet under a car running to cross the street they were about to turn onto. She yelled out to stop, which her mother did. If Jenny had not been paying attention, that little boy might have gotten very injured or worse. It pays to always be alert when you're driving.

One of the saddest days for me was when I was informed that an excellent summer student who had worked with me for two summers, died when he crossed a highway in front of a fast-moving truck and got hit. I wished I'd spent more time teaching him about horizon driving when I travelled with him. He might still be here today. He was just two weeks into his new full-time job. Too sad for words.

Another place where horizon driving is super important is around railroad tracks. Back when my mother was a young girl, she was in town when an older gent driving a horse and buggy got hit and killed by a train. Oak Lake is on the main CPR line and in those days, there wasn't much for signals at the tracks. Mum told me that she always had respect for train tracks after that day. Although she didn't actually see the train hit the horse and buggy, the memory of it stayed with her and she taught me to always pay attention around all train tracks as well.

Sadly, people are still getting hit and killed by trains. It's certainly a problem especially at level crossings in rural areas where people might go over the tracks hundreds of times when nothing is coming. But it just takes once and a few seconds of letting the guard down before tragedy strikes. It pays to horizon drive around railway tracks. And having seatbelts on is a must. Many rural folks just don't bother and it is often to their detriment. So please buckle up always.

A year ago, Bev and I heard a discussion on the radio with a person who was involved with a study having to do with why drivers often are in a collision with bicycles and motorcycles. Both seem to be invisible on the road. This person claimed that when we are driving, we actually *do* see the bike or motorbike coming, but our memory of the experience is so short that we forget we've seen them. We don't forget a semi or a school bus because of their size, but we seem to forget when it's a smaller vehicle. So, this person claimed that the proper thing to do is to say out loud, "there's a bicycle coming on my right side, I need to be cautious." The key is to say out loud or at least to yourself *See, Say, Safety*. Just the fact that you practise that slogan means you can train yourself to avoid situations that could lead you, a loved one or a stranger on a bike getting injured or worse.

When I was hauling grain during harvest the last two years, I would say to myself, *see* the possible problem, *say* what the problem might be and think *safety*. I did that when I was getting in and out of the tractor, truck or combine. Why? Because it would be so easy to miss a step and tumble to the ground if a person weren't paying 100 percent attention. Complacency is probably the cause of many accidents. Like horizon driving, it pays to be aware of the possibilities of something going wrong where you could get injured. And remember, older bones are more brittle, break easier and consequently take longer to heal.

Another area to practise good safety habits is around ladders. A friend who is a bit older had a ladder slip on ice when he was coming down from his roof in winter. He broke his pelvis. It was extremely painful but he fully recovered over time. A fellow-curler is a building contractor and he said, "You must secure a ladder any time you're going up on a roof. They're too dangerous otherwise." Someone needs to hold the ladder, or it needs to be tethered with a chain or rope, or somehow made immovable. I've heard of people having a fall when they got on a ladder that was set up in the back of a pickup truck. When the ladder moved, the person bounced off the tailgate of the truck and suffered broken ribs and other injuries. Secure your ladders, folks! We are less flexible as we get older and we need to pay attention to all these tips to avoid injury.

And for another safety precaution, for winter you can buy a pair of Yak Tracks to go under your shoes or winter boots. I wear them all winter, especially when it rains before the snow comes. Then footing underneath is treacherous. If you don't know what Yak Tracks are, then google them and you'll find many designs. You'll recognize them right away. One time I slipped very quickly on a skiff of new snow that was covering ice where I was walking. I didn't know the ice-patch was there and down I went in a nanosecond and injured my knee. The same thing happened to Bev and she banged her elbow, which took a long time to heal. Again, she went down in a split second with no time to break her fall. But I actually deter from my main message.

Horizon driving is the key to this chapter. And I would like everyone who reads this book to learn how to practise some form of this when they're driving. If possible, sign up for a defensive driving course. Learn to pay attention every time you turn the key in the ignition. What's the consequence of not paying attention? You as a very healthy person or your passengers or someone you collide with, could end up in a wheelchair or be dead. Harsh words, I know, but we all know of people who were either injured or killed because someone wasn't paying attention while driving. Please pay attention. It may save your life.

> **Horizon driving is the key to this chapter. And I would like everyone who reads this book to learn how to practise some form of this when they're driving. If possible, sign up for a defensive driving course.**

a slimmer you
TIPS FROM CHAPTER 19:

1. Horizon driving is a good habit.

2. Horizon driving saves lives.

3. Learn See, Say, Safety.

CHAPTER 20

Listen to the Music

"Music, once admitted to the soul, becomes a sort of spirit, and never dies." This is a quote by Edward Bulwer Lytton that I found on the internet. Lytton was a British writer and historian who lived from 1803 to 1873. I thought this quote quite appropriate to open this chapter on music.

But, I'm sure by now, like a few chapters in this book, you're thinking, *I thought this book was about losing weight, keeping it off, getting fit and living a healthy lifestyle. What gives?* If you want to view this book that way, that's fine, and we all have different ways of looking at things. But in the interest of the fitness and the pleasure that music brings I had to include a chapter on music. And remember, you hardly ever go to an exercise class or to a gym where music isn't playing in the background. It helps to calm the brain while exercising.

Along with music comes dance and there are numerous benefits of dancing, most of which are attached to music. So, if we agree that the two are interconnected, then we'll carry on and hopefully this chapter will explain how both music and dance work together and combine with fitness.

I want to start by telling another story about when I was young and growing up on the farm. Before I was in grade one, a once-shut-down one-room school was re-opened in our local school district. Grades 1 through 8 were taught at Harvey School but it closed permanently after my 6th Grade and we all ended up going to school in Oak Lake. But the fondest memories of that school revolved around the Christmas concerts and the dances that were held at the school. If you remember those times, then you'll know that a teacher could be judged, not only on their academic capabilities but also on their ability to design and choreograph a Christmas concert. Most were very capable of doing just that and any miniscule salary increase coming their way might depend on those capabilities. But once again, I digress.

It was at Harvey School where I learned how to dance. My parents were great dancers and they were poetry in motion as they whirled around the dance floor to music from an old up-right piano, accompanied by a fiddle. I watched them swing to polkas, old-time waltzes, fox-trots, two-steps, schottisches and of course the butterfly. There were usually three songs to a set, so if you were dancing a polka or the three-person butterfly, you were usually sweating and puffing by the time it was over. What a workout! I learned all these dances and when to swing one way or the other and how to avoid stepping on my partner's toes. I never thought anything about being able to dance, it was just a part of growing up in our family where it was another aspect of our rural upbringing.

My dad also knew most of the square dances and he called out the moves and coached many folks to learn them, as well. My siblings and I were able to catch on fairly quickly and we enjoyed the dances where our dad George happily called out the squares. You get the picture that dancing was something we did as we were growing up. Later on, I remember attending a Youth Conference in Brandon and one of the things we were taught was how to ball-room dance. I slipped into the mode very quickly and a number of girls commented about how smoothly I danced. A lot of their partners had "two left feet." In other words, they couldn't follow the moves and often stepped on their partner's toes. I was pleased to get praise from the numerous partners I danced with at that conference.

When we were dancing, we never once thought about the benefits of what we were doing. We were just dancing for fun. But now I've learned there are many health benefits tied to dancing. These include improved muscle strength and for sure muscle endurance. If you think of dancing the polka or the butterfly or if you've watched the Irish Riverdance folks you'll notice how they seem to be able to dance at a terrific pace seemingly forever. Or go online and watch the local Métis group called the Asham Stompers as they dance on stage in one of their more than ten-minute-long sets of constantly moving performances. If you don't think dancing is a workout, just pay attention to how strenuous it must be to sustain that level of dancing for so long. Heck, you'll get your own workout just by watching them.

Or watch people who are trained to perform the tango, or salsa or ballroom dances. A dream of mine would be to go to Vienna and attend a high-level ballroom dancing convention. Observing couples waltzing around the ballroom to an original Strauss Waltz tune, would be a tremendous experience. To me that would be the ultimate.

Dancing has been shown to improve flexibility and posture as well as to lift a person's spirit while they dance and afterwards. And often by attending dance lessons or joining dance groups, new friendships develop which facilitates the socialization of older adults. This is recognized as being very important for people's mental health as they age. As well, taking up waltzing after experiencing a mild to moderate heart event has been shown to improve heart health and breathing. Furthermore, it appears to have more benefits than simply pedalling a stationary bike or walking on a treadmill. There are also reports of older folks significantly reducing the amount of pain killers they take for arthritis when they've signed up for a low-impact dance program. And dancing has been shown to reduce levels of depression and anxiety.

Other studies of the benefits of dance mention increased core strength, coordination, balance, flexibility, muscle tone, weight management (*yep*), and stronger bones. And it helps people form a positive image while increasing their self-esteem. I know of groups of people, who never danced before because of religious reasons, taking up dance later in life because they realized all the benefits that can be derived from dancing. That's a solid endorsement if you ask me.

In writing this chapter, I just had to talk to a fellow fitness class attendee, Wilma Horton. When I first met Wilma and her husband Ken, they were a very fit couple. Not only did they attend fitness classes but they were also involved with a square-dancing group. For years they would go to dances all over Manitoba. "We weren't just square-dancing," said Wilma. "We also did round-dancing, pattern dancing, a lot of old-fashioned dances like foxtrots, two-steps, schottisches, waltz quadrilles, plus old-time waltzes and others."

And Wilma admitted that their favourite times of all were when they attended square-dancing jamborees. These were also held around Manitoba and in other provinces. Every two years, there was a combined jamboree where they met fellow dancers from North Dakota, Minnesota and Saskatchewan. "Not only were they a lot of fun, but we met so many other people and made life-long friendships. People we've kept in touch with over the years. It was all so much fun."

And Wilma admits that it was absolutely about fitness and more. "It certainly is beneficial to helping one stay fit, but it's also about the music, the activity, the socialization and those all-important friendships." These jamborees were not dancing competitions, they were all about getting together and having fun with food and tons of camaraderie. "And we always left a dance or a jamboree in a good frame of mind," claimed Wilma. "We never left in a bad mood because we'd always had so much fun." Wilma and Ken attended these dances for over thirty years together starting after their children were grown up. Unfortunately, Wilma lost her dance partner in December of 2019 when Ken succumbed to lung cancer just a few months short of his eighty-ninth birthday.

So now that we know of all the benefits that dancing provides, it's time to address the music that almost always accompanies dance. If it's just a fiddle and piano like at the old one-room-school dances or a full-blown orchestra like the 145-member philharmonic orchestra of Vienna, music is what makes the world go round. There are so many music genres to choose from: jazz, blues, rock and roll, classical, reggae, Cajun, or whatever you want. There are over 1,300 types of music from around the world for your listening pleasure.

Back in 1957, in my hometown of Oak Lake, Manitoba, a few teenage kids decided to form a band. And they pulled it off. They selected the name the Kool Kats and were often in demand in neighbouring towns and villages. I grew up dancing to their music and I thought they were the greatest band ever. The band originally consisted of Sharon Hatch on piano, Inez Iverson played the accordion, Ed Whitcomb and Ron Wahl played guitars and Jim Parrott played the drums.

When someone mentioned that it would be a good addition if the Kool Kats had a brass instrument, Carlyle Smith went out and bought a used alto sax from a fellow in town and taught himself how to play it. What a neat thing to do! The band played from 1958 to 1960, and quit playing when they all left to go to university. Two of them had long careers as teachers, two obtained PhDs and went on to attract international attention with their research and ended up writing books on their accomplishments. Jim Parrott became a heart surgeon who was known internationally for his knowledge and prowess in the operating room. Kool Kat Ron Wahl had a career in the military where he started and headed up a number of different bands.

But how could these teenagers have accomplished so much with their band in such a short time while attaining academic excellence? It's because they were all such high achievers. They practised at lunch time and after school and were determined to make it work. In 2006, I got the idea to honour this group and reached out to them with the idea. They all thought it would be a good project so I interviewed each of them and pulled together a small booklet about their story. In it they shared the different pathways they'd taken in life.

I was quite surprised to learn that back in the day, the Kool Kats had a repertoire of over one hundred songs. Imagine learning to play that many songs as a group of young teenagers. On July 21, 2007, at a reunion at the annual fair in Oak Lake, four members of the Kool Kats attended and played their dance music once again. Some of them hadn't seen each other for forty-seven years. For others not so long. One comment was that, "We felt like teenagers again, if only for a few days."

And I'll leave the last word about the band to Dr. Jim Parrot who couldn't make it that day but had earlier made the comment, *"Remember we were young then and on fire. There wasn't anything we couldn't or wouldn't do. Playing in bands as a quasi-musician lets you meet a lot of good people over the years. You establish good life-long friends."* Unfortunately, Dr. Parrot passed away on in October of 2016, he was 74.

When it comes to music, we were so blessed to have grown up in the era that we did. I was about 10 when Elvis really hit the scenes and was idolized by so many for so many years. Then there was the rise of Bill Haley and the Comets, Buddy Holly and the great breakthrough of the Beatles, the Who, and the Rolling Stones out of England. What a wonderful time to be alive. I danced to the old-time music of my parent's day, and then jived to the new rock and roll bands and there was the twist and all the other new dances that came along. It was easy to stay fit in those wonderful times.

Winnipeg had its own groups, with Chad Allen and the Reflections, the Guess Who (followed by BTO). Through the '60s, Winnipeg was a mecca for music in Canada. Kids flocked to community centres as live bands played the hit tunes of the day. It was exciting times for music. And then there was the rise of the various annual festivals. The Winnipeg Folk Festival which began in 1974 is one of the best and longest running folk festivals. With over 2,900 volunteers this festival (cumulatively) welcomes over 70,000 people over the four days in early July. We've attended for several years and seen many great artists both local and from all over the world. Memorable ones have been Buffy Sainte-Marie, Bruce Cockburn, Ani DeFranco, Bonnie Raitt, Matt Anderson, Stan Rogers, and more recent local acts like the Landreth Brothers. It's always a good time and, sadly, was lost to us for two years because of Covid-19.

Other festivals that are held in Winnipeg include Folklorama, which covers two weeks in August. It's the largest and longest running multicultural festival with over 400,000 people attending each year. It features dance, costumes, music and ethnic foods from around the world. There are forty pavilions or (venues) featured around the city when it's presented. The music is what makes Folklorama go, the dance provides the energy, the costumes are gorgeous and ethnic food and drink provide nourishment. It's a very fun-filled two weeks with more than one hundred and eighty bus tours that bring in more than 13,000 visitors from outside the city, many from the northern US.

And we can't forget the Festival du Voyageur, which is a ten-day celebration in St. Boniface to honour the *voyageurs* who helped open up this area of Canada. When the North West Company merged with the Hudson's Bay Company in 1821, there were six thousand voyageurs employed by these two companies. This festival is held in the dead of winter (February) and certainly helps to shake off the winter blahs for so many folks. I've danced and sung, and tapped my feet to many great bands that performed and helped folks celebrate voyageur culture. One of my favourite international bands from the past was Hadley Castille from Louisiana. His music was based on Cajun culture and his band, starting in 1980, was a featured group at the festival for eighteen years. Dancing and singing to Cajun music, which features the accordion, fiddle, the steel guitar, the triangle, the harmonica, bass guitar and the upright bass, was just so much fun. And it helped to keep me fit.

But really, this winter festival is a celebration of the Metis culture of the area and the wonderful local music is what keeps the festival going. I'm sure that many of the young artists that play at this family fun festival attended with their parents at some time and bedtimes were something to be observed the other 355 days of the year. I must say that I've shed a few pounds over the years dancing to the up-beat music at the Festival du Voyageur.

In 2020, the Festival du Voyageur welcomed over 73,500 people and slipped in just under the wire before Covid-19 shut everything down. Usually, 95,000 people from around the world attend. The 2021 festival was cancelled but organizers are planning to celebrate again starting on February 18, 2022. If the fourth wave of the pandemic hasn't shut it down again. It actually was held but it had to be scaled down because of Covid rules and regulations. Mostly held outside, it was still a good time for those who attended.

There are many festivals throughout Manitoba every year to celebrate local culture, food and music. There is the annual Country Fest in Dauphin, which features top country bands from Canada and the US, Nickel Days in Thompson, The Trappers Festival in The Pas, the Flin Flon Trout Festival, and many more too numerous to mention. Several towns celebrate their culture with agriculture fairs that include horse and cattle shows, exhibits, dances and fireworks. There are lots of activities to attend.

I have to conclude this chapter by saying that the physical part of dancing and singing and listening to music is part of a total overall experience that encompasses the whole body. It's great to help folks lose weight and get in shape while dancing, and as we've seen it's a whole-body experience. The socialization that occurs at all these festivals helps to stimulate the brain. People leave these venues happy and relationships are made that last a lifetime. That stimulation of the brain leaves no doubt about a mind-body connection. When you set out to enjoy music and you end up dancing or tapping your feet, you are just plain having fun. But your whole body is involved in making you feel good and helping you to enjoy yourself. Isn't that a healthy way to look at life? Isn't that a good way to stay in shape with a positive attitude? Isn't that a good way to help you live a longer happier life? I believe it is. I hope you agree.

And one last story about music I have to share. When I was helping my friend and neighbour from Oak Lake, Rod Cairns, harvest his crops from 2003 to 2015, I operated a good ole White 8900 combine. I always listened to Randy Bachman's wonderful Saturday night program Vinyl Tap on CBC radio. And be darned if that old combine didn't seem to run better on into the darkness when those old Rock and Roll tunes were playing. If that isn't a good testimonial to the benefits of music, I don't know what is.

And the very last words go to Lailah Gifty Akita from her book Think Great: Be Great. Lailah is a young author from Ghana who writes inspirational and insightful books about life. She writes, *"Music, brings the soul alive. Music promotes wellness and sound mind."*

Hallelujah to that!

> **"It certainly is beneficial to helping one stay fit, but it's also about the music, the activity, the socialization and those all-important friendships."**

TIPS FOR CHAPTER 20:

1. Music and dance go hand-in-hand for fitness.

2. Many music festivals keep folks moving.

3. Music promotes wellness and sound mind.

CHAPTER 21
Mental Fitness

I know the question is going to come up so I'll address it right off the snap. What does a book about losing weight and physical fitness have to do with positive mental health? The answer is quick and easy. It has *everything* to do with mental health. There's a strong mind-body connection and it's important that people understand that steps can be taken to stave off early onset of dementia and/or Alzheimer's disease. The physical and mental aspects of our lives are *so* interconnected that it's impossible to separate the two. But it wasn't always recognized or talked about. When folks were engaged at the gym with their personal trainer, I could guess that they never said to their friends, "I'm going to the gym today to work on my physical and *mental* well-being!" No, I think they'd say something like, "I'm off to the gym for my workout today." Still, in this ever-changing world and despite more information about the topic, few people acknowledge that the mental connection of going for a workout can be as important as the physical part.

A journalist, scientist, radio and TV host, and seminar host by the name of Jay Ingram, wrote a book called *The End of Memory: A Natural History of Aging and Alzheimer's*. Some of you might remember Jay Ingram. He formerly hosted Canada's national science show called "Quirks and Quarks" on CBC radio from 1979 to 1992. He went on to host a program on the Discovery Channel Canada called "Daily Planet," from 1995 to 2011. After his aforementioned book on memory loss was published in 2014, Jay Ingram was interviewed on his old program ("Quirks and Quarks") by his replacement and current host, Bob McDonald. In that interview, he admitted that even though he'd seen his mother go downhill from a struggle with Alzheimer's disease, that wasn't the reason he wrote the book. "I wrote the book because as the disease gets more and more in our faces, I think it's important for people to just understand a little bit more of the science behind it."

I clearly remember that interview from February 2015, and was curious for more information, so I got my hands on a copy of Jay's book to learn more about the science behind Alzheimer's disease. I found that there was a lot of information to wrap my head around, but I found it fascinating reading. I had to read more than one chapter over again to try to understand what he was explaining. Ingram talked about the chemical imbalance in the brain between Alzheimer's patients and those that didn't show any symptoms. It appears that normal cells in the brain are replaced by what he describes as plaques and tangles. If you've looked into this before, you'll know what Jay Ingram means. Plaques form when small protein pieces inside the brain called beta-amyloid separate and clump together. They build up and form bigger clumps called plaques. Also, a second aspect of Alzheimer's consists of an abnormal build-up of another protein called tau. This occurs inside the neurons that are responsible for the normal processes of brain function. Tau protein always exists in the neurons of the brain, but in Alzheimer's patients, chemical changes cause tau molecules to be released inside the neurons. They then attach to other tau molecules to form tangles inside the neurons.

I know this sounds very scientific and I wanted to explain it as simply as I could from my research into this topic. There is evidence that these tangles block the neurons' ability to transport information back and forth within the brain. In an Alzheimer's-affected brain, there appears to be a build-up of abnormal tau proteins and clumped beta-amyloid proteins, which cause the confusion we see in patients who suffer from the disease. There seems to be an interplay between these two renegade runaway proteins that leads to dementia.

But I did not want to rely solely on my memory of having read Jay Ingram's book back in 2015. So, I pulled up a lecture he'd given at the 2013 Banff Summer Arts Festival, entitled "The Real Brain Science of Dementia." It's a wonderful, forty-eight-minute explanation of the whole dementia topic. A good scientific mind will find it totally fascinating. If you aren't interested in the science behind it, you'll still find it fascinating if you have a curiosity about Alzheimer's or you are questioning why your loved one is suffering so much from this disease. This lecture certainly will help you to understand.

Anyway, I want to quote from near the end of Jay Ingram's presentation because it brings out some very important facts about Alzheimer's. He says, "There is a correlation between how conscientious you are, the more you persevere, the more you set your goals and finish them, the less lazy you are, the more you meet your deadlines, all that stuff, protects you against dementia."

And when it comes to ways to stave off the onset of dementia and, ultimately, Alzheimer's disease, Ingram talks about many of the exercises we know for our brain, like Sudoku, crossword puzzles, and playing games like chess or other mind games. Anything to keep our mind working and active. But he also talks about doing many of the physical activities we've mentioned before, like walking, biking, swimming, golfing, and going to the gym for resistance training. And Ingram quotes from the Ontario Brain Institute when he discusses mental and physical activities. Apparently, folks at the institute reviewed all the literature available from all the studies about Alzheimer's disease and concluded that it's very important for people to engage in *both* mental and physical exercises.

And Ingram says, "Ideally, do both forms of exercise, but if you can't do both, if you have to pick one, then *physical exercise* is the more important one to choose. It looks like forty-five minutes of good pace walking every day can prevent about 14 percent of folks from getting

Alzheimer's. You'll die of something else first." And he went on to say that 10 percent of people over sixty-five and 50 percent of people over eighty-five will get Alzheimer's disease. If this continues into the future and people live longer, Ingram predicts that health-care costs will be incalculable.

By now you'll have gathered that it pays to be mentally as well as physically fit. When I read Jay Ingram's book, it was the very first time I'd heard of the connection between the two. I started to think about it and it really made sense. If you want to stave off the onset of dementia, it does pay to have an active brain (perform activities that stimulate your brain) and keep yourself in shape by doing something as simple as walking forty-five minutes every day. That really is only twenty-two-and-a-half minutes out one way and then walking back. Not very far actually and no matter what your weight or how fast you walk, you'll find that it will help your mental and physical well-being. Doesn't that make sense?

We need mental challenges all the time and you can think of so many. Playing simple card games with the grandchildren, working at Sudoku, cribbage, chess, checkers, bridge, scrabble, hearts, Risk, Clue, Monopoly, and many more games that you know and have played. They all help to exercise the brain on one level or another. Just do it!!

One game that Bev and I play regularly is a game that she taught me. It's called Boggle and it's a simple word game where you have to find words from letters that fall at random into sixteen squares on the plastic base of the container that you shake. It comes with a three-minute timer. It's a quick game and we'll play roughly for half an hour because we alternately shake the container four times. The object is to find as many words as you can in the three minutes. Over the years, for fun we've kept track of the number of games we've played and it totals over 3,500 games and counting. Although this game isn't for everyone, we play it to help stimulate our minds and it's become so routine, we just use it to relax for a few minutes. It's like Scrabble but is much quicker to play. And it is mentally stimulating.

Boggle and other games can help delay the early onset of dementia. It works the same way as dancing, boxing, and bicycling activities assist Parkinson's sufferers. Those activities have been shown to help those who are unfortunately blessed with that frustrating neurogenerative disease. Games and problem-solving puzzles are good pastimes to mentally challenge your brain and keep it active. They may not entirely prevent you from getting dementia or Alzheimer's disease, but they may help to delay their onset. And if you combine these games with some form of physical activity, then you could delay the onset even longer. What is there to lose? Not much to lose really and everything to gain. It could mean a stable mind and a longer and happier life.

For people who like lists, I want to point out suggestions that I found from a number of sites on the internet that recommend how to help avoid the early on-set of dementia. Most of the sites offered the same suggestions and you'll see the similarities to what we've said in other chapters as well as to what's written above. But you already know how good health and fitness play a part in so many areas of our lives. Again, the mind-body connection is undeniable.

1. Regular physical exercise: (Eureka!) This is understood to be one of the best ways to stave off early-onset of dementia. When I started this book a year ago, I wasn't totally aware of this connection but now it makes so much sense.

2. Don't smoke: On some sites this is number one, on other sites it's number 3 but it doesn't matter. You're at a higher risk of getting dementia if you smoke.

3. Eat healthy foods: A balanced diet can help reduce the risk of developing dementia. And of course, as we've discussed before, a healthy diet helps reduce the risk of problems related to cancer, Type 2 diabetes, obesity, stroke, and heart disease. Don't these same issues keep showing up?

4. Reduce alcohol intake: As we get older, it should be a no-brainer to drink less alcohol. The days of binge drinking should be in the rear-view mirror. And stay there! Too much alcohol increases the chance of getting dementia. A glass of wine or beer at your evening meal doesn't hurt. Six or more glasses are not so good.

5. Exercise the mind: An active mind can help to keep dementia at bay. It's sort of like the old saying, "use it or lose it!" In this category is the suggestion that learning a new activity or a new language, can stimulate the brain to help keep dementia away. Hobbies help you stay mentally alert.

6. Manage your health problems: If you suffer from any of the previously mentioned physical illnesses, see your doctor, (health care provider) and be sure to follow all the recommendations to help you stay as healthy as possible. It will pay off in the long run.

7. Maintain an active social life: It's important to stay in touch with family and friends. It was most difficult during Covid times and we did miss all our friends from our exercise class. Hopefully by the time this book is printed, we'll be up and exercising together again. And we'll catch up on our long-missed socialization. From the sites I've looked into, it appears that this type of interaction directly helps our mental stimulation and creates a healthy mind. Go for it! And keep it up.

8. Take control: For good mental health, exercise like walking can help control depression. If you experience hearing loss, do something about it because it can have a connection to poor mental health in the future. Try to get enough sleep. All of these issues, if not attended to, can increase the risk of suffering from dementia.

It's fairly well recognized now that there is a holistic approach to medicine. More and more medical professionals try to find out more about their patients and attempt to treat the root causes of their problems as well as the immediate issues at hand. And we know that a healthy diet, regular exercise, and a brain well exercised can lead to a longer, more enjoyable life. That's what all this is about. I'm trying to show folks that how you treat your body *and* your mind can have positive or negative repercussions down the road. But you should look ahead to your future goals. Remember your grandchildren and how much you can influence their growing lives by being there for them. They want you around as long as possible with a healthy body and a healthy mind. Ensure that you do whatever you can to make that happen.

Before I conclude this chapter, I want to introduce you to Dr. Alzheimer and include information about a significant study on a number of nuns from the order called the School Sisters of Notre Dame.

Dr. Alois Alzheimer was born in Germany in 1864, and died in 1915. He was a psychiatrist and a neuropathologist who practised his profession at his clinic. But he was also a devoted researcher who cared deeply about the overall health of his patients. As part of a team, he worked hard to understand brain function and disease. From Jay Ingram's book and lecture I learned more about how Alzheimer made breakthrough discoveries about mental health.

In 1901, a woman (Auguste D.) who was suffering from severe mental problems arrived at Dr. Alzheimer's clinic. She described to Dr. Alzheimer how confused she was and, through questioning, he determined that she was suffering from a form of dementia. In reality, her memory was shot and she had become paranoid. He provided her with the best care he could, but she never improved. In fact, her dementia grew worse. When she died in 1906, Dr. Alzheimer was able to analyze her brain by shaving thin segments and examining them under a microscope. He discovered that there was a large reduction in the neurons that transmit messages to the brain. He also discovered what we now know of the plaques and tangles that are present in the brains of patients who suffer from severe dementia. Because of those discoveries made back at the turn of the last century, severely demented patients are said to have Alzheimer's disease, named after the good doctor from Germany. A reduced number of neurons in the brain plus the existence of plaques and tangles are still used today as diagnostics for dementia and Alzheimer's disease. And it appears that around three-quarters of patients who suffer from dementia end up with Alzheimer's disease.

According to Jay Ingram in his Banff lecture, in the early 1990s, a study was conducted on 678 nuns from different convents of the School Sisters of Notre Dame in the US. These women were over seventy years of age at the time. The study (now called the Religious Order Study) followed these nuns to their death. Nuns were chosen because they all lived the same lifestyle. (Researchers wanted to study a homogeneous population.) Brains of deceased nuns were carefully examined and those who had developed Alzheimer's disease had plaques and tangles as you'd expect. What wasn't expected was that some of the nuns had many plaques and tangles but didn't show symptoms of dementia. So, the researchers dug deeper into what might have happened.

They found that all of these women, at the age of twenty-two, had to write an essay about why they wanted to enter the convent. The essays were rated for *idea density*. The more ideas that a future nun wrote about, the higher would be her "idea density." A few simple sentences rated one applicant a 3.9, which was considered to be a fairly low score. A score of 8.6 on the scale was deemed to be on the high side, meaning that the respondent had come up with more ideas. These idea densities were termed *brain reserve*. The higher her brain reserve, the better the nun was able to stave off dementia in her later years. In fact, one nun, Sister Mary, lived to be 101. However, when her brain was examined, it was found to be full of plaques and tangles. Based on that discovery, it was obvious that she was a candidate for Alzheimer's disease.

But the interesting fact was that Sister Mary did not display signs of dementia. It was baffling to the researchers because from what they'd observed in her brain, they estimated she would have a brain reserve of around four. In fact, they discovered that Sister Mary had a brain reserve of twenty-seven. Her active brain was able to counteract the devastating level of plaques and tangles and she lived a long, normal life. Recommendations from this study are to encourage folks to get a good education and be active throughout life, exercising the brain as well as the body. You want to develop and hang on to as much brain reserve as you possibly can, because you never know what the future holds.

In June 2021, a drug called Aduhelm received accelerated approval (by the Food and Drug Administration) for treating Alzheimer's disease in the US. At a price tag of US $56,000 per patient per year, for now it would be out of reach for most people. Documentation for this drug was submitted to Health Canada and they reviewed the information in order to consider its approval for Canadian patients. (I've since heard that it was not approved for use in Canada.) It's not a wonder drug however and there is still lots to be learned about its effectiveness as a treatment for Alzheimer's disease.

Brian Bethune, writing about dementia for *Maclean's* magazine in 2015, stated, "The financial burden is already enormous. The value of unpaid dementia care provided by families is at least $50 billion (now $60 b) annually in the US, as measured by income forgone by family members taking time off work and well over $100 billion (now $250 b), when measured by what a family would have paid professional caregivers. The situation is proportionate in Canada. In both countries, the cost is more than financial. For almost a decade, Statistics Canada has reported that more than half of those caring for elderly relatives confess to feelings of exhaustion and depression. And Bethune goes on to state that you can't "escape the personal toll of a sickness that is as emotionally draining as any, for those watching from the outside or looking to their own futures."

In that article, Bethune quoted Jay Ingram as saying, "Same old advice as for your health in general, pay attention to diet, especially in regard to sugar and get some form of exercise." And Bethune continued, "Solo TV watching correlates dangerously with developing Alzheimer's but social watching—say, gathering for the big game—points in the opposite direction. Bingo, in fact, may trump chess. And gossip—a source of social bonding and intense cerebral activity, with roots stretching back to primate days—may be the best. All part of the mystery of human life."

Who knew all that? It obviously pays to be socially active. Most of us *are* socially active at some level but getting a reminder is not a bad idea. Make sure your relatives who live alone see you once in a while or at least hear from you. For this book, I don't have any statistics on the harm caused by Covid-19, but we know there was a toll on mental health just from the isolation that went on for so long with so many folks. Especially the elderly.

I'm trying to show folks that how you treat your body and your mind can have positive or negative repercussions down the road.

TIPS FOR CHAPTER 21:

1. Plaques and tangles cause problems in the brain.

2. Jay Ingram's presentation explains dementia.

3. Being fit can help stave off dementia.

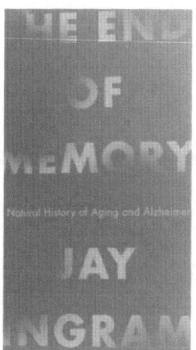

CHAPTER 22
Compressed Morbidity

Now here is a term that many of you might not have heard before. I was also in the dark until it was so aptly described by my friend, the retired Dr. Richard Blouw. We've quoted him before and he introduced me to this very good concept about how folks live their lives. The term refers to the respective outcomes of different lifestyles. I'll let Dr. Blouw explain.

"For at least four decades, while I was working as a physician, I would go to Mayo Clinic in Minnesota, for 'refresher courses' (through continuing medical education), in order to keep my head above the educational waters. One year, a lecture title 'Compression of Morbidity' was presented. At the time my friends and I didn't really understand what it would be about.

"Very shortly after the lecturer started speaking, we caught on to what he was getting at. He started out by describing two neighbours, both men in their thirties—one who was reasonably slim, exercised, didn't smoke, drank modestly, and paid attention to his health. His neighbour, on the other hand, was a pack-a-day smoker, was obese, ate a lot of fast foods and junk food, and drank excessively in a binge fashion on a weekly basis. And his exercise consisted of pushing the buttons on his TV remote. At thirty-five years of age, this obese fellow had high blood pressure, at forty, he developed early diabetes, at forty-two, he had his first heart attack; at forty-six, he had the beginnings of emphysema, at fifty-one, he had a small stroke due to his carotid artery being clogged, at fifty-five, he required bypass surgery for continuing heart disease, and at fifty-nine, he had an aortic aneurysm repair. At sixty-two, he had a partial lung removed for lung cancer, and more problems until he finally succumbed at around the age seventy. So, this poor man had, for most of his adult life, a series of operations, medications, hospitalizations, disability, and pain, and he died a relatively early death.

"His neighbour, on the other hand, the slim, active guy, had been able to avoid almost all of that, and was active into his older years, hiking in the mountains with his wife, going on canoe trips with friends and family, dancing at his grandkids' weddings, and so on. Then, at around age eighty-four, he developed some nasty disease that was relatively unfixable, and he died six months later.

"Getting back to the title of the lecture, what this man did is he compressed his illness (morbidity) into the last little bit of his life, rather than spreading it throughout almost all his life. He had a great quality of life. Most of us don't want to live to the age of Methuselah, but we want *life in our years* more than *years in our life*. And although there are no guarantees, this is the benefit of having a healthy lifestyle, which of course includes exercise."

So, isn't that a great explanation of *compressed morbidity*? When you follow what Dr. Blouw is saying, you realize that quality of life is so important. And he continued, saying that, "some of the benefits of exercise include: reduced levels of diabetes, reduced levels of dementia, decreased risk of hip fracture, lower levels of arthritis in the knee and hip with fewer replacement surgeries, less anxiety and depression, less fatigue, lower blood pressure, reduced risk of certain cancers, better sleep, less heart disease, and (above all) an improved *quality of life!*" What a list! It definitely is an endorsement for exercise. And as a family physician for so many years, Dr. Blouw certainly saw it all.

And he had more to add: "I also learned at Mayo Clinic about a US cardiologist from the 1950s, Dr. Paul Dudley White of Harvard University, who wrote the definitive textbook on heart disease that students of medicine from all over the world studied. He was also the heart physician for people like President Dwight Eisenhower. White lived in the era before we knew much about cholesterol, or the link between smoking and heart disease, before stents and artificial heart valves were invented. But he was an abundantly observant man who had a very simple adage for his patients, which was *'Eat less, walk more, and sleep more.'* This is still as true today as it was seventy years ago."

I began this book by sharing with you how I lost weight by eating all the same foods I ever ate and how I simply just started eating less of them at every meal. At the time, I didn't know of Dr. White, but here he was recommending the same thing that is the premise of this book. Dr. White and Jackrabbit Johannsen both knew that, for a good, healthy life, one of the most important things you can do is eat less. *"Push back from the table when you feel you could still eat more."* Dr. White lived to the age of eighty-seven and, if you remember from earlier in the book, Jackrabbit Johannsen lived to be 111 years old.

So, compressed morbidity was certainly a factor in both of their lives and they lived life to the fullest. We're all going to die and we never know when, but isn't it better to get the most out of every day by being as healthy as we can be, with a positive attitude? It's great to be able to stare down so many of the diseases that caused the problems for the fellow who didn't get to experience compressed morbidity. What a miserable life the poor guy had! You feel sorry for him on the one hand but you have to remember, he did have choices. And the choices he made did not help him live a healthy, happy, pain-free life.

I want you to pause for a moment and think about the choices that you can make to live the best life possible. I started by pushing back from the table when I felt I could still eat more. Everyone around you will be so grateful if you become *A Slimmer You*—a healthier you. Plan to follow the Nike slogan and *"Just do it!"*

a slimmer you

When I'm out walking the dog or riding my bike or just walking somewhere, I'm always glad to see other folks up off the couch and out there. But we do notice that runners or fellow walkers have ear-pods in and are listening to something as they walk, jog, or make their way on the path or trail we are on. When I'm out there especially early in the morning, it's nice to smell the morning dew, and in the spring the flowers that might be in bloom, along with the lilacs and fruit trees, but it's also great to hear what's out there. If you learn to appreciate nature, you'll hear birds of all kinds calling to each other or using their mating calls. Geese, gulls, robins, chickadees, finches, meadowlarks (outside the city limits), owls, mourning doves, kestrels, marlins, and, around a lake, loons and grebes, crows and ravens. There is lots to hear, every day.

When my oldest daughter Laura was very young, we would listen to the chickadee's mating call and we always said it sounded like it was calling out "cheeseburger." Hearing the sounds of nature is so fun and rewarding, I always feel people are missing so much of the pleasure of being out for a walk if they aren't hearing the sounds, seeing the sights, or smelling what nature has to offer. Now maybe the odour of skunk isn't so sweet, but if you're out in nature, you learn to accept whatever is there. The senses are sharp in the morning and there is so much to see, hear, and smell. Try it if you haven't done it lately. It's invigorating.

Why am I bringing all this up and how does it relate to life? It's because of the death of a wonderful man, Jim Henderson, who was Senior Stick of the 1969 agriculture degree program, my graduating year. He was someone I admired for his ability to just get things done. You might say I was envious because I seemed to have very little of the talent he displayed. Later, even though he was suffering terribly from his struggles with Parkinson's Disease, Jim made the effort and was able to attend the fiftieth reunion of our graduation from agriculture in Winnipeg, in July 2019. Sadly, he passed away on June 22, 2021.

But I want you to read what his wife Liz so kindly wrote about Jim's life with Parkinson's disease.

"Although exercise is important for us all, it takes on even greater importance in Parkinson's, given the physical changes associated with the disease. Exercise can improve one's physical body, improve endurance, improve one's general well-being, and help delay or reduce the problems of Parkinson's.

"He had always been active in sports but Jim was never one to go to the gym or be involved in an exercise program. All that changed when he was diagnosed with Parkinson's. At first, he could still golf and curl, but then he decided to attend the CRIS clinic (Community Rehabilitation Interdisciplinary Service). There, he worked with a number of specialists. He ended up going to stick curling, and eventually had to give up golfing.

"When Jim fell off his treadmill, we replaced it with a recumbent stationary bike, which was much easier for him to use. He then went to a gym for exercise classes geared to those with Parkinson's and the one activity that he enjoyed most was boxing. At first, he was in a boxing class but then he worked one-on-one with a trainer. Boxing is good both physically and mentally for those dealing with Parkinson's. Other sufferers find enjoyment from tai chi, yoga, dancing, or cycling.

"When Covid hit and gyms were forced to close, Jim lost ground in many ways. He really missed the boxing classes. It was difficult to get him to do things on his own at home, even though the Parkinson's Association of Alberta put many ideas and programs on their website.

"Gradually, it became more and more difficult to do things and even walking was a challenge. Before he died, Jim was confined to a wheelchair. However, I do believe that exercise was a great help in delaying some of his symptoms."

Dr. Judy Anderson, professor emerita and former Head of the department of biological sciences in the faculty of science at the University of Manitoba has some insights into the value of our exercise classes. She was also a prof in the department of human anatomy and cell science. As a fellow fitness class member Judy was willing to share her thoughts about what those classes meant to her.

"I grew up as a pretty active person, although not what I'd call athletic. However, over the years, my husband and I found that our professional careers dominated most of our waking hours. Once he retired my husband Jay started to attend fitness classes three mornings a week at the university where I worked. Over time he started to look good and claimed that he felt better than when he was working.

"My work as a professor included teaching and my research interest is skeletal muscle—the muscle that allows us to move voluntarily, talk, sing, lift, jump, hike, dance, and exercise. In particular, I studied muscle regeneration and muscle diseases. I knew from reading the research literature how important physical activity is for overall function and quality of life; I knew it *for sure* and talked about it in presentations and lectures to my students! I just didn't find—or, rather, MAKE—time to ensure that I maintained my own physical capabilities.

"After hearing my husband talk about his workouts over a few years, I signed up for the exercise class. When I could, I attended classes and found that the many benefits I derived from those workouts was way better than sitting at my desk five mornings a week.

"The instructor, Sharon Couldwell, took us through initial warm-up, then a little more deliberate with the warm-up stretching and muscle movements. Then we'd go to our mats and begin the pattern of exercises, resistance exercises with weights and tasks that moved the big muscles first, and eventually she got us to exercise the smaller muscles. We alternated exercises for upper and lower limbs, flexion and extension of muscles, crossing the different joints, core, and peripheral muscle groups. Our pattern of exercises ended with a cool-down stretch to calmer music.

"But most importantly, people in the class became friends and when you do something together with friends, it's definitely good for your health. And, besides, where else might I have been able to walk a kilometre on a Wednesday morning and chat with an economist, a farmer, an engineer, a teacher, a nurse, a dentist, a social worker, or an artist, and ask a question or answer one of theirs?"

And Judy continued, "One day, I broke my leg in a slip-on-the-ice accident. It was a bad break that needed surgery and lots of internal hardware and I was truly laid up for three months. But inside that cast, I started exercising and really took physiotherapy sessions to heart during rehabilitation. I was back in the fitness class just after I stopped using the crutches. I gradually regained a lot of balance and strength, and I got even stronger than before that accident.

As the years progressed, I actually developed what I could see were muscles under the skin—muscle definition in body-building. Me, an academic, with muscles! My husband and I noticed that shirts and pants fit differently, and I felt different inside, too (in a good way).

Sharon sadly has now retired and the pandemic ended the classes, but we do miss the exercises and camaraderie that are so much a part of the fitness class.

But I know I MUST get going again. I'm still strong, but know that my resistance to fatigue, power, and balance have all declined to some degree over the past year due to the gyms and exercise classes being shut down. So, I have to get back at it.

Now, first, warm up, then squats, now push-ups, then quadriceps flexion and knee extension, then biceps, glutes, deltoids . . . living anatomy is fun after all!"

For the last few words of this chapter, I want to take you back to the lecture that Jay Ingram gave at the Banff Centre of the Arts. He ended by talking about when it comes to brain reserve, people who are destined for Alzheimer's just simply have nothing left. Ingram says there's a tipping point where some people start to decline earlier than others. But other folks hang on longer and then decline quickly, only to end up at the same level as those in the first group. But it's like compressed morbidity, which we talked about earlier in this chapter. Ingram suggests that it's better to hang on as long as one can before suffering from the disease. We know that crossword puzzles, Sudoku, board games, etc., can help delay the onset of dementia, but, again, Ingram quotes the Ontario Brain Institute as stating that the best way to delay the onset of the disease is by becoming and staying fit.

Becoming fit can help your body in so many ways. When you know how fitness relates to compressed morbidity and also to possibly delaying the onset of dementia, even if you are genetically predisposed to getting it, then shouldn't it make sense to get up off the couch and get moving? Your family will appreciate it, you'll create more memories with your grandchildren, and, best of all, it's important for your own quality of life. Is there any reason for you not to get up and go for a forty-five-minute walk? You can start today. Good luck!

We're all going to die and we never know when, but isn't it better to get the most out of every day by being as healthy as we can be, with a positive attitude.

TIPS FROM CHAPTER 22:

1. Aim for as healthy a life as you can.

2. Exercise benefits the body and the mind.

3. It's all about quality of life.

CHAPTER 23

The Other Side of the Coin

I've tried not to be judgemental in this book and I don't want to sound preachy but I believe this chapter has to be written. The information presented here is readily available and I believe that some people won't like reading the facts. But I think it's necessary to point out that certain habits can lead to people contracting diseases and possibly dying too early. They leave behind grieving families and children and grandchildren who miss them so dearly. So, what am I talking about? I'm talking about health problems that are defined by cancers, by diabetes and by heart and stroke events. There are many more diseases out there but for this chapter, I want to concentrate on this group because they are often at the forefront of continuing health problems.

Cancer: Believe it or not, according to information printed by the Canadian Cancer Society, smoking is still the main culprit behind many health issues, especially as it relates to lung cancer. Even though smoking rates have dropped dramatically since governments realized the harm that smoking does and introduced the so-called sin tax on cigarettes, it's still a major cause of cancers. The Canadian Cancer Society claims that smoking is the cause of 30 percent of fatal cancers in Canada and of course is a major cause of lung cancer.

It wasn't very long ago that smoking was so accepted generally, that there were ash-trays on every third seat at meetings and conferences. Smoking in offices was accepted. Heck, there was even a smoking section at the back of airplanes and in certain areas of restaurants. I remember getting a last-minute standing-room-only ticket to watch the Winnipeg game of the Summit Series between Russia and Canada in 1972. I was in the rafters of the old arena. I was excited, the atmosphere was electric and the game ended in a four-four tie. But one of the things I clearly remember from that game was the blue haze that hung above the playing surface. There were so many people smoking in the arena at the time, that you might have thought it would be difficult for the players to breathe. But they concentrated on the game and put on a fantastic display of hockey skills. Thank goodness smoking is not allowed inside public places like that anymore.

As an aside to that, 37 percent of Canadians smoked in 1970. That was reduced by half by 2011 and more recently it got down to close to 13 percent but I've read that it is creeping up again. Too bad, and I guess there are many reasons for that happening. Vaping might be one reason for the increase.

Another cause of a high percentage of cancers can be traced to poor diet. The Canadian Cancer Society reports that 20 percent of fatal cancers can be traced back to folks who are overweight. That means that a total of 50 percent or half of fatal cancers in Canada are claimed to be due to smoking and/or poor diet.

In our own province, CancerCare Manitoba ran banner ads in the Winnipeg Free Press that stated "You can reduce your risk of cancer by 50 percent." If you go to *protectyourtomorrow.ca* you'll find important information on how to do this. They also report that, "Every year about 1,000 Manitobans are diagnosed with a cancer related to an unhealthy diet and another 400 of all cancers diagnosed annually in Manitobans are weight-related. And that annually 800 Manitobans die, earlier than they might have, because they smoked at one time or were exposed to second-hand smoke."

CancerCare strongly recommends that people adopt a healthier, balanced diet to help reduce the incidence of many cancer types. And they want people to regularly visit their doctor or health care professional and dentist. CancerCare also claims that "being active is important to staying healthy and maintaining a healthy body weight."

Where have you heard all this before? I share this information because it really is the key to a longer, healthier life. And that's exactly what I want for anyone who might be reading this book. CancerCare folks caution that an active lifestyle doesn't mean running a marathon or spending hours at the gym. They recommend that "you walk once a day or take the stairs instead of the elevator. Reduce the time in front of the television or computer. Play actively with your kids. Walk or ride a bicycle for short trips or use nearby walking and cycling paths." These are all great tips for a healthy lifestyle, tips that we've mentioned a number of times in this book. It becomes a theme after a while, doesn't it? But I truly believe it makes sense and I hope that you, too, will see the pattern and accept it for your own philosophy on life.

CancerCare Manitoba claims that, "Regular exercise can reduce your risk of colon cancer and may also reduce your risk of breast cancer. It can also reduce stress, increase energy levels and improve your outlook on life."

In a *Reader's Digest* article from 2010, I read how women can reduce their risk of dying from breast cancer by 33 percent by changing from a sedentary lifestyle to a moderately active one. This was according to a University of South Carolina study, where they claim that "Just thirty minutes a day walking (moderate fitness) is all you need." For more up-to-date information, check the internet to compare the results from different sources. There appears to be validity to the claim, although the numbers do vary.

And from the Canadian Cancer society it was estimated that there were almost 226,000 cases in 2020 and over 83,000 deaths from cancer in Canada. The report claims that cancer is the leading cause of death and is responsible for 30 percent of all deaths, as previously stated.

Diabetes: Again, there is much written about diabetes and how it affects people's health. You can look up information online, but I'll briefly mention some of what I discovered.

The definition of diabetes is as follows: *Diabetes is a disease that occurs when your blood glucose, also called blood sugar, is too high. Blood glucose is your main source of energy and comes from the food you eat.*

Embracing a healthy lifestyle can help people manage health issues associated with diabetes. If a person is overweight, it's hard for them to manage Type 2 diabetes. There is also a risk of having high cholesterol and high blood pressure. So, when diabetics decide to adopt a healthy diet, they need to *"control portion sizes and learn to read food labels in order to help maintain a proper weight. It is important to limit carbohydrates that are found in foods like table sugar, cake, soda pop, candy, and jellies."* Recommendations found in the Canada Food Guide can help people make healthier choices when it comes to filling their grocery carts.

One woman who was diagnosed with Type 2 diabetes was a busy person, often working fourteen-to-sixteen-hour days and not eating proper meals. Her comment was, "When I ate at work, I didn't make good food choices. Then I decided that no matter how much I loved to eat unhealthy foods, it wasn't worth dying for, and it was time to make a change." (1)

I know those changes are not easy, but you have to make up your mind that you want to do it, develop a plan, and stick to it.

Another woman from North Carolina, who was diagnosed with Type 2 diabetes, said she learned to make a few small changes to her favourite recipes that allowed her to continue to eat her cherished southern dishes. Before she made those changes, she claims that her favourite home-cooked meals were *unfortunately* unhealthy. (1)

Physical activity: A very overweight person who loses 7 percent of their body fat, can reduce their risk of developing diabetes by around a half. That's an astounding figure and the risk is even further reduced if more weight is lost. Some form of exercise is required.

After devising a weight-loss plan with your doctor, you can work with local gym instructors who will recommend proper workouts that are appropriate for your body size. You can choose to hire a personal trainer to help you develop a program that is right for you. The main issue here is for you to make a decision to do something.

One man with diabetes decided to walk for ten minutes a day in order to get active and lose weight. Then he decided to add one more minute a day. In a year he got up to sixty minutes a day, every day, and he lost 139 pounds. Remarkable, yes, but it was his determination to live a healthier lifestyle that saw him through. (1)

Dr. Richard Nesto, who is the chairman of the Department of Cardiovascular Medicine at Lahey Clinic Medical Center in Burlington, Mass., and a professor of medicine at Tufts University School of Medicine, cautions people about diabetes. "Most people don't understand that having diabetes means they are two to four times more likely to suffer a heart attack or stroke. Add in smoking and that risk is multiplied. The earlier you can quit smoking once you've been diagnosed with diabetes, the better your chances of preventing coronary artery disease and other deadly complications."

It's also important to manage stress levels if you've been diagnosed with diabetes. Stress causes different responses in different people but it can trigger aches and pains including headaches and lead to unhealthy choices like overeating, drinking too much alcohol, procrastination and lack of sleep. Most folks can handle a bit of stress in their lives but they need to learn to deal with it in a healthy way.

Heart attack and stroke prevention: Again, you can look up information you need to know about preventing heart attacks or strokes. The information is all available. But in order to help you become more aware, I want to outline some of the changes that can help you make good choices when it comes to good heart health.

First up, is once again a recommendation that people need to quit smoking if they smoke. It's not an easy thing to do, but it's much tougher on the body to recover from a heart attack or stroke or to live with chronic heart disease. And learning to eat a healthy diet is mentioned next. This is reported to be one of the best ways to fight against cardiovascular disease. The food you eat and the amount can affect other risk factors that lead to poor heart health. So, it's important to choose nutrient-rich foods (which contain vitamins, minerals and fibres and are lower in calories) over nutrient-poor foods that contain a high number of calories.

Also, it's important to manage your cholesterol levels. If fat is lodged in your arteries, sooner or later it could lead to a heart attack or stroke. My doctor, Dr. Saggid Hashmi, is always careful to check my blood levels of LDL cholesterol (bad cholesterol) and HDL cholesterol (good cholesterol). He says that the best medicine to prescribe is to "lower your levels of LDL cholesterol and increase the levels of HDL cholesterol."

High levels of LDL cholesterol result in a build-up of a fatty plaque-like substance that forms on the walls of blood vessels. At too high a level the natural flow of blood becomes blocked and there is a dangerous risk of a heart attack or stroke. A steady diet of food that contains trans-fats will cause LDL levels to rise.

HDL cholesterol helps to remove other forms of harmful cholesterol (like LDL) from the bloodstream. If HDL levels in the blood are too low there is a greater risk of heart disease. Smoking, being overweight and living a sedentary lifestyle all contribute to low HDL levels in the blood. As do diets that are high in refined carbohydrates (eg: white bread, sugar).

A normal *blood pressure* to aim for is 120/80. That's a relatively safe and optimal level to attain. If it's much higher than that, a person might be heading toward a stroke. If your doctor says you need medication for high BP, take their advice. But it's possible to set a goal to reduce prescription requirements by starting to lose weight slowly and incorporating simple exercises like walking. It's all about lifestyle. And you do have a choice.

And another theme (that we've heard before) from the heart and stroke folks is to initiate some physical activity. They state once again that, "Research has shown that 150 minutes per week of moderate-intensity physical activity can help lower blood pressure, lower cholesterol levels and keep your weight at a healthy level. If you've been inactive, start out slowly. Even a few minutes at a time can result in health benefits. Studies show that people who have achieved even a moderate level of fitness are much less likely to die *early* than those with a low fitness level."

Isn't that exactly what this book is all about? I know that if you're reading this, you'll know that I wish for you to be around longer for your children and your grandchildren. They'll love you dearly if you choose to get up off the couch and do something to improve your chances of living longer. And the best news is that you can start today by getting out and going for a short walk. Just be like that fellow who started slowly, added a minute a day and lost 139 pounds in one year: a slow and healthy way to lose weight. And I'll bet he is now able to do his hour long walk every day with more of a sprightly step compared to when he first started out.

We have a neighbour Dave Smith who goes for a 3.6-kilometre (2.25-mile) walk every morning around 6 a.m. He's eighty-four years old with not an ounce of fat on his body. He goes for that walk summer and winter and never lets poor weather or cold weather be an excuse for not taking that walk. Dave doesn't take any prescription drugs and says that years ago a doctor told him that he could live to an old age with the help of prescription drugs or if he decided to stay *fit*, he could live to an old age without those prescriptions. He happily chose the latter lifestyle.

And a fellow, Rene Ammann who attends our church is an avid bicycle rider. He rides a bicycle 3-5 days a week in the summer and 3-4 days a week in the winter. He covers over 8,000 kms every year so over the last 5 years he has ridden enough to circumnavigate the globe. He is 78 and has no intention of slowing down. And of course, he is in phenomenal shape.

Dave Smith and I are indeed very fortunate in not having to take prescription drugs. Many people have health problems that can only be remedied with the help of prescription drugs. And what about folks who suffer from chronic pain or those recovering from operations, or those waiting for hip or knee replacements? Without the interventions of their prescription drugs, they would probably suffer through a lot more pain. "Better Living Through Chemistry" is a take-off on an old advertising slogan of the chemical company Dupont. It certainly makes sense when you know the number of people who have been helped by prescription drugs.

The heart and stroke folks want you to aim for a healthy weight for your body. They claim that, "obesity is prevalent in our society and not just for adults but for children as well. Fad diets and supplements are not the answer. Good nutrition, controlling calorie intake and physical activity are the only way to maintain a healthy weight."

There, it's not just little ole me saying this over and over again. A group that knows the dangers of being overweight are sending a message as well. And they go on to say, "Obesity places you at risk for high cholesterol levels, high blood pressure and insulin resistance, a precursor of type 2 diabetes ---- the very factors that heighten your risk of cardiovascular disease. Remember that your BMI reading can help to tell you whether or not your weight is healthy."

Also, these good folks want you to limit your alcohol intake. Their caution is that, drinking too much alcohol can raise blood pressure, increase the incidence of cardiomyopathy (diseases of the heart muscle), stroke and cancer. And it can contribute to irregular heartbeats. Excessive alcohol consumption can contribute to obesity, alcoholism, suicide, broken homes and accidents.

Here, I have to share a true story about myself. Not too long ago, my wife Bev, myself, and our friend Bill Forsyth were at our cabin in the northwest region of Ontario. It was a fine day and a gin and tonic seemed to be just the right thing to have in the late afternoon. It went down smoothly and quickly. So, it wasn't long before one quick drink led to four in a fairly short period of time. When I was asked to help prepare supper, I gladly grabbed a paring knife to do some fine chopping and within half a minute I'd sliced into a finger. Not to the bone, thank goodness, but there was a fair amount of blood. So, I learned the negative consequences of too many drinks in a short period of time. At my age, I should have known better. Right?

Most people have heard that moderate alcohol consumption can have positive effects on the heart, but that knowledge comes with a precaution. "If you do drink alcohol, then you need to limit your consumption to no more than two drinks a day for men and no more than one drink a day for women." Those levels might help protect your heart but they don't lead to the other problems we've just listed above. It's definitely not recommended that non-drinkers start drinking alcohol (for heart health purposes) or that drinkers increase the amount they already drink. And we all know that you *can't* tell young people that binge drinking every weekend might catch up to them later in life. Especially if they don't have an active lifestyle. I know because I was one of those people back in the day. It's just what we did. I can't tell you why. It was a popular social thing to do back then. As it still is now.

Getting outside and moving is not only a healthy lifestyle choice, but it helps with a person's mental attitude. That's because you meet folks you've seen numerous times before and, although you might not be good friends, you'll get a smile and some cheerful dialogue. This was true even during Covid-restricted times. Maybe it's even more important now. We find that almost all the people we meet are very pleasant. You know how that can set the tone and mood for the whole day? To say nothing of the wildlife we might see and the wonderful birdsongs we hear. No ear-pods for us, as we want to hear whatever sounds there might be waiting for us as we stroll leisurely through the woods, forest-bathing all the way.

Collectively, I think it's important to think of the costs to our health-care system that come from people needing to visit a doctor regularly. Or of folks who require numerous prescription drugs in order to keep going. The costs are astronomical. The Canadian Institute for Health Information (CIHI) suggests that health-care costs $264 billion every year and that, of course, continues to rise. That figure equates to $7,068 for each Canadian citizen. I love our *socialized* medical system and we are told by many (who don't know) that our health-care system is free. It's not free because every person or corporation who pays taxes in this country shares in its cost. Our governments over the years have made sure the system works. You know that our wonderful health-care system will only be sustainable if everyone does their part to eat healthy foods, pay attention to their body weight, and get moving even a little bit.

Do you think that now is the time for you to start moving? Everyone knows of a loved one they've lost who should still be here. That's sad to no longer have a spouse, a father, a mother, a brother, a sister, a nephew, niece, uncle, aunt, grandfather or grandmother who could still be with us if they had just made better life choices for themselves. Luckily, wonderful memories and pictures help us to remember them.

When I read the obituaries and the stories of different people's lives, I love reading about older folks who have lived a long and healthy life. They are all role models to me. But there are so many I read about who have died far too early and when there are requests to donate in their honour, it's often to the heart and stroke foundation, or to the cancer society or to the diabetes foundation. I find it so very sad and I think, *"If only that sixty-five-year-old or fifty-five-year-old (or whatever age) had changed their lifestyle a wee bit, maybe they would still be with us today, playing with their grandchildren and watching them grow up to be fine citizens."*

Covid really has made this whole picture quite a bit worse. As I edit this in January 2022, the death toll since the beginning of the pandemic, in Canada, is over 31,000 deaths. (Over 5.5 million worldwide). Sadly, many of those folks died alone in hospitals or in nursing homes because their families, of course, were not allowed to visit them. Others passed away because they had other compromising health conditions. In other words, the healthier your body is, the better you are able to ward off attacks by diseases or viruses like Covid-19. It's entirely up to you to choose how you want to live your life. I just know that the choices you make for a healthier lifestyle will make your family happy and you'll look and feel better, too. Go for it!!!

(1) These stories are from an American Heart Association website. All information was reviewed by editorial staff and by science and medicine advisors.

CancerCare claims that "Being active is important to staying healthy and helping to maintain a healthy body weight."

TIPS FROM CHAPTER 23:

1. A healthy body is better able to fight off tough diseases.

2. Good nutrition and fitness are desirable goals.

3. Walking is a cheap and easy way to good health.

CHAPTER 24

IF

I met a good friend, Malcolm McEachern, from Carman, Manitoba, when we studied agriculture at the University of Manitoba in the mid-1960s. Not long after I met him, he told me that his father had strongly encouraged him to memorize the poem "IF," by Rudyard Kipling. Written in 1896 and published in 1910, the poem lays out in explicit detail how people should live their lives. I was impressed when Malcolm could easily reel off the whole poem, a poem I'd never heard of before. And the advice from the poem is as relevant today as it was in 1896. If not more so. And because *If* is the title for this last chapter, I feel it's appropriate to present the poem here:

IF

By Rudyard Kipling

If you can keep your head when all about you

Are losing theirs and blaming it on you,

If you can trust yourself when all men doubt you,

But make allowance for their doubting too;

If you can wait and not be tired by waiting,

Or being lied about, don't deal in lies,

Or being hated, don't give way to hating,

And yet don't look too good, nor talk too wise:

LARRY GOMPF

If you can dream—and not make dreams your master;

If you can think—and not make thoughts your aim;

If you can meet with Triumph and Disaster

And treat those two impostors just the same;

If you can bear to hear the truth you've spoken

Twisted by knaves to make a trap for fools,

Or watch the things you gave your life to, broken,

And stoop and build 'em up with worn-out tools:

If you can make one heap of all your winnings

And risk it on one turn of pitch-and-toss,

And lose, and start again at your beginnings

And never breathe a word about your loss;

If you can force your heart and nerve and sinew

To serve your turn long after they are gone,

And so hold on when there is nothing in you

Except the Will which says to them: 'Hold on!'

If you can talk with crowds and keep your virtue,

Or walk with Kings—nor lose the common touch,

If neither foes nor loving friends can hurt you,

If all men count with you, but none too much;

If you can fill the unforgiving minute

With sixty seconds' worth of distance run,

Yours is the Earth and everything that's in it,

And—which is more—you'll be a Man, my son!

a slimmer you

This message is so strong that *if* folks the world over could bring themselves to practise these words, wouldn't it be a better place to live? At least the poem points out that it's important to look at life with a positive attitude.

I've gone back through the chapters from this book to search for content for this last one. This quote is from the very first chapter I wrote, *"If* you are serious about losing weight and *if* you have the desire and the will power to do it, then I know that reducing portion size is the place to start." And I really mean it. You'll never start a weight-loss trend (without being on some type of diet, of course) *if* you don't start eating a bit less. In other words, push away from the table when you think you could still eat more.

And once again, *if* you do make the conscious effort to start to lose weight by eating less, then it makes sense to attempt to become a little more fit. I don't mean you have to become a gym-rat in order to be fit. Throughout this book I talk about getting up off the couch and starting to move as a good beginning. You've heard from both Dr. Richard Blouw and Dr. Judy Anderson of the importance of being fit—Dr. Blouw from what he's seen during his years as a physician and Dr. Anderson from the benefits of being in our fitness class.

If you want to be able to bend over and tie your shoelaces or shovel snow or do anything athletic without your back *going out*, then you'll want your core to be as strong as it can be. And ensuring a strong core takes discipline and requires a certain level of fitness. It doesn't happen overnight—but in time it can become stronger.

And for me personally, once I decided to lose weight in the most natural way I could think of (and to also continue to eat all the foods I've always enjoyed), I realized that losing weight *slowly* was the only way to go. I'm fairly certain that *if* I had not chosen to go that route then this book would not be in your hands today. *If* I'd followed some fad diet, I believe I would have lost weight, yes, but I truly believe those lost pounds would most likely have found their way back again and there would be no story to tell.

But lest you think I'm painting myself as a pure perfect picture of health, you might remember that I promised to share with you a few of my physical imperfections. So here goes.

I tolerate a disease called tinnitus. For those who might not know, it's a ringing in the ears. It can be in one ear or the other, but in my case it's both ears. One day more than a dozen years ago, I woke up and the ringing was there. My doctor sent me to a specialist (for a second opinion) and, basically, I was told that there was nothing that could be done, so I learned to live with it. *If* I had the ability, I would just wish that ringing to go away. But of course, as you know, I can't just wave the magic wand and have tinnitus disappear.

I call the noise "the dancing girls in my head." Sometimes they dance louder than at other times, but they're always there dancing away. The cause, well, it might be because I rode on open-air tractors and combines when I was younger. That's the most probable explanation, but it may not be the definitive answer. And it's always interesting when talking to different friends or acquaintances when I discover that they are sufferers as well. And they didn't all drive open-air noisy machines either.

Another problem I have is that one morning a few years ago, I woke up to discover that I had blurred vision in the lower left quadrant of my right eye. My young optometrist sent me to a specialist and she ran several tests. Sure enough, something had caused the blur in my vision, but there was no explanation as to what. However, the good news is that if I look straight ahead, my vision is not impaired in any way, shape, or form. So, I'm grateful for that. *If* I could wish that minor inconvenience away, then I would get rid of it, as well.

Also, I clamp my teeth tightly when I'm sleeping (bruxism) and I don't know how many teeth I've had to have restored or removed because of this nasty habit. I need to wear an "appliance" on my lower teeth to prevent more tooth damage. Why do I clamp down on my teeth? I just don't know, but it's a fact. Probably some mental angst somewhere in my brain. Again, *if* only.

And my sleeping habits aren't the greatest, even though throughout this book I've mentioned several times that older folks need to get a good night's sleep for a long and healthy life. I get up to use the washroom and, more often than not, I'm not able to get back to sleep. So, I'll read the newspaper, watch something I've recorded on TV, or do a Sudoku or crossword until I get tired again and fall asleep in my recliner. I don't like this interrupted sleep habit and *if* I had my druthers, I'd sleep right through or at least will myself to get back to sleep. But for me, it is what it is.

And as mentioned before, I have a weakness for chocolate. I feel I need to have chocolate-covered peanut M&M's and chocolate-covered almonds in the house at all times. I can control how many I eat of one or the other during a given day. *If* I didn't have a certain degree of self-control, or *if* I weren't weighing myself every day, then I might gain back all the weight I've worked so hard to get rid of. I always claim that I don't get my caffeine fix from coffee; I get it from chocolate.

Again, *if* you truly want to shed some pounds and get more fit in the most natural way, you may choose to follow some or all of the guidelines mentioned in this book—guidelines that helped me reach my weight-loss goals. Push away from the table when you feel you could still eat more, control the portion size with smaller plates, and eat only one serving. Use the scales daily to monitor the trend of your weight, up or down. And for sure get active in one way or another. There are so many activities that a person can do to develop a healthier lifestyle and one of them is to get up and get moving. As Dr. Blouw has said, walking forty-five minutes a day is a good target to start with. It will help shed pounds and you'll be on your way to looking and feeling good. Isn't that the best way to respond to your own statement, "*If* I could only lose some weight and keep it off"?

If you want to change your eating habits, remember to select wholesome and nutritious food. Don't constantly rely on processed foods or fast foods to round out your dietary choices. No longer is there a need to spend hours canning vegetables and fruit, like our mothers and grandmothers had to do, in order to make it through the winters. The food industry makes these readily available to us on the grocery shelves. Check labels closely to choose low sodium food that is stored in water not in juice or syrup.

Fresh fruits and veggies are available all year round. It's great. But in season, nothing compares to locally grown fresh produce. Take advantage of your farmers' markets. Not only will you meet some very interesting farm people, you'll get the freshest fruit and vegetables that you can buy. And you'll support your local economy. Think about the 100-mile diet. In season, nothing beats it.

And for store-bought food, remember that it's important to learn to read labels so you aren't consuming too much salt, sugar, and/or fat all the time. Processed food can do us in *if* we eat too much of it on a daily basis. Forget that it might be cheaper. Re-read the chapters on salt, sugar, and fat, and *if* you want more information on how the big companies adjust ingredients to give you that flavour burst or get you to your bliss point, read Michael Moss's book of the same title, Salt Sugar Fat. That book could help you change your eating habits for the better.

If there weren't so many brands of sugary drinks on offer now, then people wouldn't be consuming so many "empty" calories every day. The selection ranges in the hundreds and each one has varied amounts of sugar in it. And most are way too sweet. When I was a kid, it was a treat to get a soda pop. Now kids can have one or more every day. *If* their consumption was not monitored (and, for many, it isn't), they could be heading toward obesity at a young age. We see that on a number of kids on the street every day. And as we've discussed several times, that could lead to future problems like: joint issues, diabetes, heart and stroke events, cancer, and an overall lower quality of life or even death at too early an age.

We've talked about the value of a dog in this book. Not everyone can or should own a dog and it's naïve to suggest it. But I'd like to point out that there are some wonderful service dogs working in the community to help many disabled people function in their neighbourhood. And *if* you'd like a clear understanding of the value of a dog, the next time you visit someone in a children's hospital, a personal care home or an assisted living place, take a look at any visiting dogs and see for yourself the joy that they bring. The instant smiles on the faces of most of those folks are immeasurable.

If you want to protect yourself from an untimely death or crippling injury, make sure to take the time to learn and practise *horizon driving*. It's so easy to do and it's like insurance for when you're behind the wheel. When you hear of people getting wiped out in a collision, a number of times it's because the driver of a vehicle drove across the median lane and ran smack into another vehicle. So, be constantly aware of what's going on around you.

And you might be surprised to learn that Canada has the *second* highest percentage of deaths per capita caused by drunk drivers in the world. In first place is South Africa. Canada has nearly 1,500 people killed and over 60,000 people injured annually from drivers who get behind the wheel after drinking alcohol. *If* only we had the means to absolutely stop this from happening.

And the numbers don't totally add up but I've checked the internet and found that there are another 400 people killed in Canada from inattention of people texting while driving and the same number from people who fall asleep at the wheel. *If* drivers could only get it through their heads that they are six times more likely to cause an accident *if* they are talking on their cell phone while driving, and *twenty-three times* more likely *if* they are texting, then maybe more lives could be saved every year. Please, drivers, pay attention and put your phones down while driving or pull over *if* that call or text just has to be made or taken. *If* you do, then you and others might stay alive and continue to live a longer, fuller life.

And from the chapter on music and dance, I just have to share this story. Back when my mother-in-law Jean Jamieson was recovering from a stroke and waiting for a room in a nursing home, she was placed on a ward in the Misericordia Hospital in Winnipeg, and on that ward was the meanest, snarkiest woman you could ever encounter. She grumbled and complained in a mean voice almost every day. She struck out at her health-care workers and fellow patients. People like my mother-in-law always had to give her a wide berth. There were no smiles and she glared at health-care workers as *if* it was their fault that she was in the hospital. Most of the time, the dear soul's mind was somewhere else and for sure not close by. She was perpetually angry.

But once in a while one of the nurses would squeeze in enough time to get this lady up to dance to music that was playing in the hallway. Well, you should have seen her smile and she could dance beautifully. And sometimes she would sing along to a tune she recognized from her youth. She had a beautiful singing voice. That young girl of her past was deep in that mind somewhere. It's just that no one saw or heard that youngster very often. The woman would quickly return to her old, miserable, irascible self and be totally unkind to everyone around her. *If* only there was more money available to hire care workers to be with people like her a lot more, then their lives and the lives of folks around them would undoubtedly be less miserable.

There are more *ifs* that I could write from this book but I won't drag it out any longer and risk losing your attention. However, I do have a couple of requests. *If* you can manage to squeeze in the time, google up the video titled the *Old Man Practises Lifting a Kettle Bell Weight*. It's less than three minutes long but it does show the essence of what I've been trying to point out as you've read about my level of fitness. You'll not be disappointed.

And *if* you're interested to learn more about mental health and the mysteries around plaques and tangles in the brain, call up Jay Ingram's video of his presentation at the Banff Centre of the Arts, entitled "The Real Brain Science of Dementia." It's forty-eight minutes long but Ingram does an excellent job of explaining what goes on in the brain of someone who suffers from dementia. And what continues to happen as many of them sadly transition into the depths of Alzheimer's disease.

If you childless folks who've been reading this book and learning the steps to take to get in shape are thinking that the advice is only for people with children and grandchildren, then I want to assure you that this advice is for you, as well. *If* you have a circle of friends who like to participate in different activities, you might want to get in shape to keep up with them. *If* you like to travel to exotic locations, go hunting or fishing in remote areas, or just generally walk the trails nearby, I believe that any one of those activities will be easier *if* you manage to lose extra weight that you are currently carrying around. Don't do it for me, or for anyone else; do it for yourself. I know you'll feel better and you'll look better, as well.

a slimmer you

And *if* you pay attention to the discussion on fitness as it relates to compressed morbidity and mental health, doesn't it make sense to want to live a healthier and happier life? There really is no downside to any of this. You'll be living a fuller life and you'll enjoy it a lot more.

If you truly want to shed some pounds and get more fit in the most natural way, you may choose to follow some or all of the guidelines that helped me reach my weight-loss goals.

TIPS FROM CHAPTER 24:

1. Read again the poem "IF" by Rudyard Kipling.

2. If you can, make changes that will make a difference.

3. If you want a longer, healthier life, work at getting fit.

The answer to the skill testing question on page 114 is 70 years old. How close were you?

AFTERWORD:

More facts about issues surrounding heart and stroke were provided by Alison Davis, senior associate manager for Heart and Stroke Canada:

- Nine in ten people in Canada have at least one risk factor for heart disease, stroke, and vascular cognitive impairment.[32]
- Eight in ten cases (or 80 percent) of premature heart disease and stroke are preventable through healthy lifestyle behaviours.[33]
- 70 percent of people in Canada do not eat enough fruits and vegetables.[34]
- People in Canada get almost 50 percent of their daily calories from ultra-processed foods.[35]
- Youth vaping rates are increasing.[36,37] Vaping may raise the risk of heart disease and stroke.[38,39]

---

32. Public Health Agency of Canada. *Tracking Heart Disease and Stroke in Canada*. 2009. https://www.phac-aspc.gc.ca/publicat/2009/cvd-avc/pdf/cvd-avs-2009-eng.pdf
33. Chiuve SE, Rexrode KM, Spiegelman D, Logroscino G, Manson JE, Rimm EB. "Primary prevention of stroke by healthy lifestyle." *Circulation*. 2008;118(9):947-954. doi:10.1161/CIRCULATIONAHA.108.781062; Chiuve SE, McCullough ML, Sacks FM, Rimm EB. Healthy lifestyle factors in the primary prevention of coronary heart disease among men: benefits among users and nonusers of lipid-lowering and antihypertensive medications. *Circulation*. 2006;114(2):160-167. doi:10.1161/CIRCULATIONAHA.106.621417; Stampfer MJ, Hu FB, Manson JE, Rimm EB, Willett WC. Primary prevention of coronary heart disease in women through diet and lifestyle. *N Engl J Med*. 2000;343(1):16-22. doi:10.1056/NEJM200007063430103.
34. Government of Canada SC. Fruit and vegetable consumption, 2016. https://www150.statcan.gc.ca/n1/pub/82-625-x/2017001/article/54860-eng.htm. Published September 27, 2017. Accessed December 14, 2018.
35. Government of Canada SC. Nutrient intakes from food, 2015. https://www150.statcan.gc.ca/n1/pub/82-625-x/2017001/article/14830-eng.htm. Published June 20, 2017. Accessed June 13, 2019.
36. Canada H. Canadian Student Tobacco, Alcohol and Drugs Survey. aem. https://www.canada.ca/en/health-canada/services/canadian-student-tobacco-alcohol-drugs-survey.html. Published September 27, 2019. Accessed November 25, 2019.
37. Hammond D, Reid JL, Rynard VL, et al. Prevalence of vaping and smoking among adolescents in Canada, England, and the United States: repeat national cross-sectional surveys. BMJ. 2019; 365: l2219. doi:10.1136/bmj.l2219
38. Glantz SA, Bareham DW. E-Cigarettes: Use, Effects on Smoking, Risks, and Policy Implications. Annu Rev Public Health. 2018;39(1):215-235. doi:10.1146/annurev-publhealth-040617-013757
39. Alzahrani T, Pena I, Temesgen N, Glantz SA. Association Between Electronic Cigarette Use and Myocardial Infarction. Am J Prev Med. 2018;55(4):455-461. doi:10.1016/j.amepre.2018.05.004

Acknowledgements and thanks go to the following folks, who definitely helped in the creation of this book.

To my wife, Bev, who encouraged and supported me throughout this whole journey and carefully read every word of every chapter more than once and offered wonderful advice and suggestions for needed changes.

To my daughters, Laura, Sarah, Michelle, and Jenny and their spouses for encouragement along the way as I lost weight and for their unending support for this project as it progressed.

To my book coach, Les Kletke, whose support, enthusiasm, and positive attitude kept me on track through all the steps of the way. His coaching and encouragement were indeed invaluable.

A special shout-out to Sharon Couldwell, who started me on my fitness journey and, through encouragement and kind words, kept me going. She also willingly contributed to the book.

To Dr. Richard Blouw, Dr. Judy Anderson, Wilma Horton, Liz Henderson, my nephew Tim Gompf, my sister-in-law Monica Gompf, my neighbour Dave Smith, and Rene Ammann all who were interviewed and contributed to the success of *A Slimmer You*.

To my friend Jim Ellis whose photo was directly responsible for jolting me into doing something about the extra weight I was carrying around my belly.

To my son-in-law Steve Melo who was forthcoming with his information about how drinking soda pop every day was negatively affecting his health.

To my nephews Tyler and Kirby Gompf, who have been positive influencers for a number of years, encouraging me with comments like, "You can do it!" "Go for it!" or "Just do it!"

To many friends, acquaintances, and even a few strangers who were so supportive of this endeavour. Their enthusiasm of this project helped to keep me going.

To Michael Moss (*Salt Sugar Fat*) and to Jay Ingram (*The End of Memory*), who both gave me permission to use material and quotes from their respective books.

To my sister Marlene, brother Karl, and their spouses, and to sister-in-law Nora for moral support during the creation of the manuscript.

To the Bartmanovich family of Glenlea, Manitoba, who annually give me the opportunity to indulge in something I love to do: being out in their fields and helping to get their grain in the bin.

To everyone at FriesenPress who had a hand in making this book a reality, especially to Emily Perkins, Meaghan McClur and Renzel Villegas who were so encouraging and who kept me focused and kept the process moving along.

To our wonderful springer spaniel dogs, first Taylor and now Coco, who, for twenty-five years now, have gotten us out for two walks a day through rain, snow, sleet, sunny, cold and/or windy weather, and kept us going.

And lastly to my wonderful eleven grandchildren, who were happy to pose for the picture and who were all very supportive of this book.

ABOUT THE AUTHOR

Larry Gompf grew up on a farm and pursued a career in agriculture. After successfully achieving his target weight, Larry's next goal is to share what he's learned with others. Larry loves his healthy lifestyle, and he wants to help others create healthy lifestyles that they too can love.

Larry lives in Winnipeg, Manitoba with his wife, Bev, and their dog, Coco. They love to visit their cabin in northwest Ontario, to enjoy boating, fishing, and spending time with their eleven grandchildren in the great outdoors.

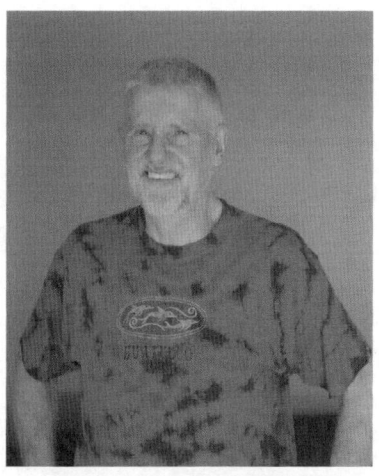

Printed in Canada